Books by Mayer Eisenstein, M.D., J.D., M.P.H.

Home Birth Advantage
Safer Medicine
Don't Vaccinate Before You Educate

Medical Disclaimer

UNAVOIDABLY DANGEROUS contains the opinions, based on scientific fact and evidence, of its author, Mayer Eisenstein, M.D., J.D., M.P.H. It is not intended to replace the advice of your physician or healthcare provider. If any reader requires personal medical attention, a competent medical professional should be consulted. The author and publisher disclaim any responsibility for any liability, loss or risk, personal or otherwise, which is incurred as a consequence, directly or indirectly, by the use and application of any of the contents of this book.

Unavoidably Dangerous

Medical Hazards of Synthetic

HRT

Hormone Replacement Therapy

Mayer Eisenstein, M.D., J.D., M.P.H.

UNAVOIDABLY DANGEROUS

MEDICAL HAZARDS OF SYNTHETIC HRT

Hormone Replacement Therapy

Mayer Eisenstein, M.D., J.D., M.P.H.

Published by CMI Press
http://www.homefirst.com

ISBN 0-9670444-4-8 $16.95

Printed in the United States of America

TABLE OF CONTENTS

FOREWORD

I Think - Therefore I Believe

Physicians' attitudes towards medical procedures and treatments have been greatly influenced by their belief systems. If a physician believes something is right, all the scientific studies will not sway his/her thinking. The overwhelming scientific evidence documenting the dangers of synthetic HRT has not convinced many physicians to stop prescribing Prempro™, Premarin®, etc. (see page 123). When obstetricians were surveyed with a hypothetical question, "If it is proven that it is 100% safe to deliver a baby vaginally after a previously cesarean section what would you do?" 80% answered they would still do another cesarean section. When questioned about their response, even though the hypothesis stated that it is 100% safe to deliver vaginally after cesarean, their answer was "I do not believe that it is possible." A similar survey was conducted regarding episiotomy. The hypothesis given is that episiotomy is proven to be 100% unnecessary. 80% of physicians surveyed responded they would still perform episiotomies because they believed that episiotomies are necessary.

I was very bothered by these studies because the implication is that even if scientific studies were conducted and even if the results of these studies unequivocally confirmed my hypothesis regarding the dangers of the HRT and the Pill, as well as the safety of home birth, infant feeding, etc. there would be no change in physician behavior.

I asked a theologian, "Why would learned professional physicians not practice medicine in accordance with the evidence based scientific studies?" He was not surprised by the findings that I presented to him. He related to me a similar study that he had read. A hypothetical question was posed to people. "If you had the following two choices in life...

1) you and your family would be financially poor all your life, but happy every minute of your life, or

2) you and your family would be financially wealthy all your life, but depressed every minute.

You would not be able to change either scenario regardless what you did. Which option would you choose?" 80% of the people surveyed chose option two - the money. when asked why, they said because they could not believe that with all the money in the world they would not be happy. "You see," the theologian said to me, "Attitudes and beliefs, many times, supercede evidence to the contrary."

My belief is that if myths can destroy reality, why not make reality destroy the myth? We are facing a very difficult situation in medicine. I am bringing my arguments directly to you, the individual who is affected by these procedures, pills, vaccines, etc. in order to give you the ability to say "No" to many unscientific medical procedures. Is the answer to abandon modern medicine? NO, the answer is for medicine to follow the results of the scientific studies which have already been conducted.

INTRODUCTION

Sometimes an answer is so simple it escapes everyone. More than 20,000,000 women today take some form of **synthetic** HRT (hormone replacement therapy) risking increased breast cancer, ovarian cancer, stroke, blood clots, and no reduction in heart disease, gallbladder disease and atherosclerosis. I use the word **SYNTHETIC** because the HRT drugs that women take have estrogenic and progestational activity, but they are **not "bio-identical"** to human estrogens and progesterone. Bioidentical [see page 1] means that the chemical structure is **"identical"** to that hormone which is found in the human body. There is not even one structural difference, no matter how small, between the molecules. Anyone who has ever studied chemistry or biochemistry understands that even the change of one element in a complex biochemical structure can drastically alter its function. Any minute molecular change can alter the molecule's effect on the body and can also alter metabolic pathways leading to undesirable changes. The difference between testosterone, a masculinizing hormone, and estradiol (one of the body's natural estrogens), a feminizing hormone, is ONE ELEMENT, so seemingly insignificant that at first glance they look exactly the same, but the difference speaks for itself. *See page 8*

These synthetic hormones do help with menopausal symptoms, i.e. hot flashes, night sweats, vaginal dryness, etc. Does this mean that women must suffer with pre and menopausal symptoms, if they were to stop taking these unavoidably dangerous hormones? No, many women have no menopausal symptoms and they will do fine without any hormonal treatment, natural or synthetic. Some women will do fine with lifestyle changes, i.e. low carbohydrate diet, exercise, etc. Over 90% of women who have menopausal symptoms will greatly benefit from a simple, safe (bio-identical) product - natural progesterone cream (NPC). I have treated over 3,000 women with NPC with incredible success. Why is this such a well kept secret? The answer goes back to physicians belief vs. scientific evidence. In *UNAVOIDABLY DANGEROUS,* I bring you the scientific evidence explaining why the synthetic hormones are unavoidably dangerous. I bring you excerpts from the "Women's Health Initiative Study" (WHI), sponsored by the National Institute of Health (NIH), which in the summer of 2002, after five years of study, stopped short of completing their study of Prempro™ [synthetic, conjugated estrogen and synthetic progesterone]. They found that the incidence of: 1) breast cancer; 2) ovarian cancer; 3) blood clots; and 4) heart disease; in the synthetic HRT group far exceeded that of the control group, and decided it was too dangerous to continue. I outline the link between estrogen and breast cancer while presenting excerpts from the National Toxicology Program (NTP - a division of NIH) whose committee has recommended that steroidal estrogens be placed on the cancer list for the "10th RoC" (Report on Carcinogens). I then outline programs for safer alternatives for women with menopausal symptoms, i.e. hot flashes, night sweats, vaginal dryness, etc. Will these programs work for everyone? No, but they will work for more than 90% of hormone related problems. What should you do? Start by familiarizing yourself with the complex and confusing medical language of hormone replacement therapy by going to the Definition of HRT Terms (see page 1). If you are presently taking any synthetic HRT, read this book and go to my website: www.homefirst.com.

Definition of HRT Terms

bio-identical

Bio-identical hormones have the same chemical structure as hormones that are made by the human body. The term "bio-identical" does not indicate the source of the hormone, but rather indicates that the chemical structure of the replacement hormone is identical to that of the hormone naturally found in the human body. In order for a replacement hormone to fully replicate the function of hormones which were originally naturally produced and present in the human body, the chemical structure must exactly match the original. Bio-identical hormones are able to follow normal metabolic pathways so that essential active metabolites are formed in response to hormone replacement therapy.

carcinogens

Substances that increase the risk of abnormal growths, neoplasms, in humans or animals.

diethylstilbestrol (DES)

A synthetic drug with estrogenic like activity, today would be described as a SERM (designer estrogen). DES was originally prescribed to prevent miscarriage. DES did not prevent miscarriage but it did cause malformation of the reproductive organs in some offspring who were exposed to the drug while in utero.

equilin

A naturally (for horses - not humans) occurring steroid with estrogenic activity obtained from the urine of pregnant mares, not bio-identical to any one of the three human estrogens.

estrogen

The term "estrogen" actually refers to a group of related female steroid sexual hormones, each with a unique profile of activity. Under normal circumstances, a woman's circulating estrogen levels fluctuate based on her menstrual cycle. The three main estrogens produced in female humans are:

- Estrone - E1 - (10-20% of circulating estrogens) is the primary estrogen produced after menopause.
- Estradiol - E2 - (10-30% of circulating estrogens) is the most potent and major secretory product of the ovary, and the predominant estrogen produced before menopause.
- Estriol - E3 - (60-80% of circulating estrogens) a metabolite of estradiol and usually the predominant estrogenic metabolite in urine. During pregnancy, large amounts of estriol are produced by the placenta.

estrogen receptor

Cytoplasmic proteins that bind estrogens and migrate to the nucleus where they regulate DNA transcription. Evaluation of the state of estrogen receptors in breast cancer patients has become clinically important and determines the likelihood of response to anti-estrogen therapy.

estrogenic

Having an action similar to that of an estrogen.

estrogens, conjugated (Premarin®)

An estrogenic compound formed by the union of seven different estrogens obtained from urine of pregnant mares. The principal estrogen present is sodium estrone sulfate. The total estrogenic potency of the preparation is expressed in terms of an equivalent quantity of sodium estrone sulfate.

From the PDR

Premarin® (conjugated estrogens tablets, USP) for oral administration contains a mixture of estrogens obtained exclusively from natural sources (natural to horses, not natural to humans), occurring as the sodium salts of water-soluble estrogen sulfates blended to represent the average composition of material derived from pregnant mares' urine. It is a mixture of sodium estrone sulfate and sodium equilin sulfate. It contains as concomitant components, as sodium sulfate conjugates, 17 (alpha)-dihydroequilin, 17 (alpha)-estradiol, and 17 (beta)-dihydroequilin.

estrogens, synthetic

Compounds obtained by chemical synthesis which possess estrogenic activity, but differ in molecular structure (they are not bio-identical) from naturally occurring estrogens. They may be derived from horses (Premarin®, Prempro™) or from plant substances.

natural

Occurs in nature. Although it occurs in nature - may not be natural to a certain species, i.e. equilin, one of the horse estrogens is natural for horses but not natural to humans.

phyto-estrogen

A group name for plants that have estrogenic like activity, i.e. soy.

Prempro™

PREMPRO™ consists of conjugated estrogens found in Premarin® tablets and medroxyprogesterone acetate (MPA) for oral administration.

> The conjugated estrogens found in Premarin® tablets are a mixture of sodium estrone sulfate and sodium equilin [horse estrogen - natural to horses not humans] sulfate. They contain as concomitant compo-

nents, as sodium sulfate conjugates, 17 (alpha)-dihydroequilin, 17 (alpha)-estradiol and 17 (beta)-dihydroequilin.

Medroxyprogesterone is a synthetic progesterone.

progestational hormones, synthetic

Compounds obtained by chemical synthesis that possess progestational activity, but differ in structure from naturally occurring progestational hormones.

progesterone

Produced in the corpus luteum, as an antagonist of estrogens. Promotes proliferation of uterine mucosa and the implantation of the developing fetus, prevents further follicular development.

progesterone receptor

Cytoplasmic proteins that bind progesterones and migrate to the nucleus where they regulate DNA transcription. Evaluation of the state of progesterone receptors in breast cancer patients has become clinically important and determines the likelihood of response to progesterone therapy.

progestin

Generic term for any substance, natural or synthetic, that effects some or all of the biological changes produced by progesterone.

SERM [Selective Estrogen Receptor Modulator]

(Also known as designer estrogens) A new class of drugs which possess some, but not all, of the actions of estrogens. SERMs are not steriodal estrogens. For example, raloxifene (Evista®) is classified as a SERM because it allegedly prevents bone loss (like estrogen) and allegedly lowers serum cholesterol (like estrogen) but (unlike estrogen) does not allegedly stimulate the endometrial lining of the uterus.

steroidal estrogens

A group name for estrogens that contain a hydrogenated cyclopentanoperhydrophenanthrene ring system. Some of the substances are naturally occurring and others are synthetic.

steroidogenesis

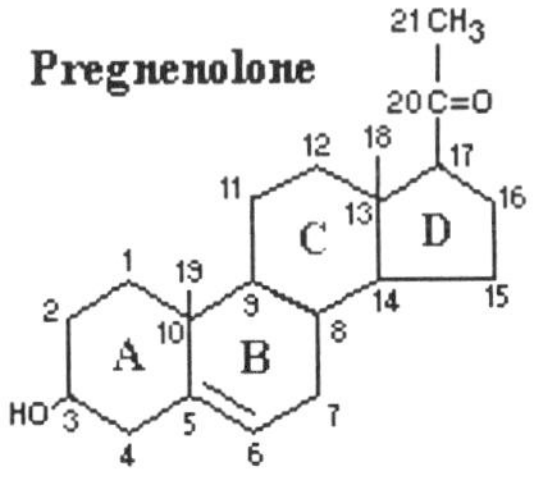

Steroid hormones are derivatives of cholesterol and are synthesized by a variety of tissues, most prominently the adrenal gland and gonads. The basic cyclopentanoperhydrophenanthrene ring (the A B C D rings) structure and carbon numbering system of all steroid hormones is depicted to the right, using pregnenolone as an example.

xeno-estrogen

A completely synthetic chemical compound, which exerts estrogenic-like activity, i.e. PCBs and DDTs, which do not naturally occur in nature and believed to be resistant to environmental degradation.

CHAPTER I

SYNTHETIC HORMONE REPLACEMENT THERAPY *UNAVOIDABLY DANGEROUS*

Did nature make American women deficient in estrogen and progesterone? Does every American woman need synthetic chemical estrogen or progesterone chemicals when they reach menopause? Do synthetic hormones protect women from heart disease and osteoporosis? Is a synthetic hormone, which is structurally different, better than a natural hormone? Must every phase of our lives become a condition that must be treated with chemical drugs?

WHAT ARE SYNTHETIC HORMONES ??

The pharmaceutical companies that create synthetic hormones are brilliant. They have ingeniously developed synthetic estrogen and progesterone compounds which, in many ways, mimic the body's own estrogens and progesterone. The problem is that these compounds are not bio-identical [see page 1] in chemical structure to human estrogens or progesterone. In order to patent their designer synthetic estrogen and progestin products, the pharmaceutical companies must alter the natural chemical structure. These altered synthetic chemicals have been linked to many serious side-effects including but not limited to high blood pressure, blood clots in the lung, brain, headaches, changes in libido, fatigue, hirsutism, hemorrhagic eruptions, coagulation problems (a partial listing from the PDR [Physicians Desk Reference]). Hormones are messengers which instruct different cells in our body to perform various tasks. By taking exogenous (introduced from or produced outside the human body) hormones we are able to give the body instructions that the body would not normally give itself. By taking synthetic estrogen and synthetic progesterone during one's reproductive life, messages are sent telling the body not to ovulate or not to let the fertilized egg implant into the uterus. Use of these hormones can lessen or eliminate pre-menopausal and menopausal symptoms. The question is what price are we paying for these alleged benefits? Are there other, safer means available?

The Price of Synthetic Hormones

Increased risk for blood clots, stroke, and cancer are just a part of the price that we are paying for ingesting synthetic hormones. But why? The hormone messengers that our body produces are very specific. Even a small alteration in the hormone's structure can bring about a completely different message. The difference in the structure between estradiol (one of the body's natural estrogens - see

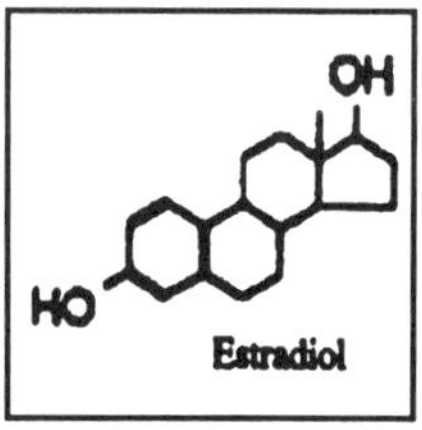

Figure 1

Estradiol - one of the body's natural estrogens.

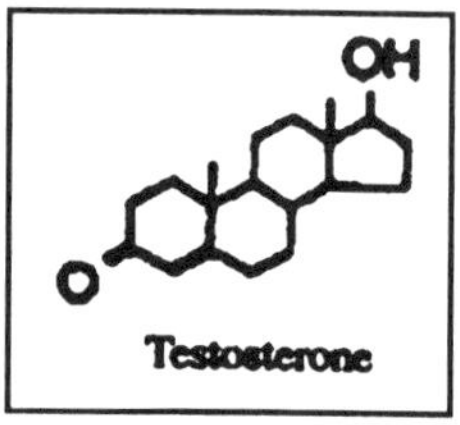

Figure 2

Natural testosterone.

Figure 1) and testosterone (see Figure 2), is seemingly very little. The difference is the HO attachment to estradiol vs. the O attachment to testosterone on the bottom of the hormone molecule. Yet, we know that the production of estradiol by the body will cause feminization and the production of testosterone will cause masculinization.

The synthetic hormones sold by the drug companies (see Fig. 3) are structurally similar to those produced by the body and will produce estrogenic and progestational effects.

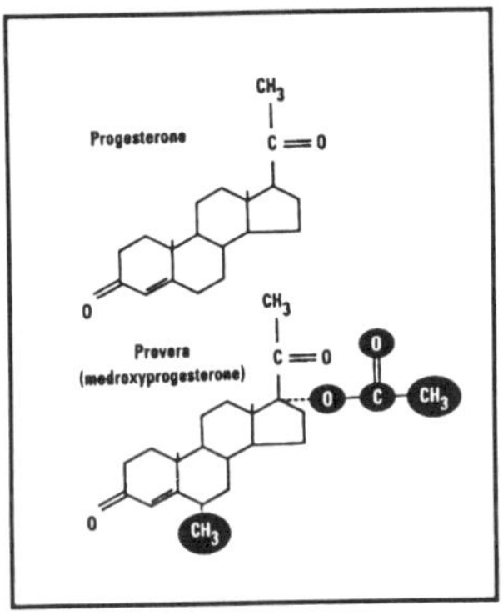

Figure 3

Note the similarity between natural progesterone and Provera® (one of the synthetic progestins).

However, they are not the same. The synthetic hormones are capable of producing other effects as mentioned above. The structural alteration is necessary because these synthetic compounds, if not structurally altered, would not exert their effect in a "pill" form. They would be broken down by the body or the effect would be too short lived to be effective. Bioidentical natural estrogen and bioidentical natural progesterone can be produced in cream forms which can be readily absorbed; however, they cannot be patented. This makes them less desirable to the pharmaceutical companies, from a monetary standpoint.

We have 50 years of history with the synthetic estrogen-like compound Diethylstilbestrol or DES (see page 1). In the 1950's doctors prescribed the synthetic estrogen-like drug, DES, to pregnant women to prevent miscarriages. Leading researchers and gynecologists hailed the man-made synthetic estrogen-like DES, as a wonder drug with a host of potential uses. Almost immediately, researchers began prescribing DES for women who were experiencing problems during pregnancy, in the belief that insufficient estrogen levels caused miscarriage and premature births.

In the decades that followed, doctors not only prescribed DES to prevent miscarriages, they began to recommend it also for untroubled pregnancies, as if it were a vitamin that could improve on nature. This would prove to be a massive human experiment.

In 1971, a rare vaginal cancer began being diagnosed in young women. This cancer was linked to the very drug their mothers had taken to prevent miscarriages, the synthetic estrogenic-like compound DES. Until this connection was made, most scientists believed that the placenta acted as a barrier, letting good substances in and keeping bad substances out. Physicians believed that drugs could be safely administered during pregnancy, unless they saw immediate problems or obvious birth defects, because of their mistaken belief in the "placental barrier". The most painful aspect of the DES tragedy is that the drug did not even prevent miscarriages.

Those who took DES did not have fewer miscarriages, fewer premature babies, or fewer infant deaths. The drug, DES, not only did not prevent miscarriages, but, increased the risk of malformation and cancer of the urogenital tract (vagina, cervix, ovaries, testes) in the children born to these women.

This tragic and unintended experiment demonstrated that chemicals could cross the placenta, disrupt the development of the baby, and have serious effects that might not be evident until decades later.

The DES experience offered another critical lesson as well, that is relevant not just to those exposed to DES, but to all of us. The developmental effects of DES made it clear that the human body could mistake a man made chemical (i.e. birth control pill, hormone replacement therapy) for a (nature made) hormone. DES was taken off the market subsequently and labeled as "known to be a human carcinogen".

In 1943, Willard Allen, a scientist working at the University of Washington, St. Louis, extracted an estrogenic product from the urine of a pregnant mare. This proved to be inexpensive and easy to obtain. It also had fewer side effects than some of the earlier hormones extracted from animals. The patents for the "horse urine estrogen" were sold to Ayerst Laboratories. Premarin® (**Pr**egnant **ma**re's u**rin**e) quickly gained dominance in the market.

Premarin® (conjugated estrogen see page 2) is formed by the blending and union of several of the different estrogens obtained from the pregnant mare urine. Many of the estrogens in this blend are specific to horses and not found in humans. Approximately 75% of "horse estrogen urine" is estrone, a hormone that is also produced by human females, but as a much lower percentage of total estrogen. However, horses also excrete approximately 40 other forms of estrogen into their urine. These horse estrogen hormones are not bio-identical - or biologically equivalent - to the other two main types of estrogen - estriol and estradiol - that occur naturally in women. Drs. Whitehead and Campbell, two leading menopause researchers in England, did studies of the potencies of the different types of estrogens and the effects of the various horse estrogens on different target organs in the body. They showed that conjugated equine estrogens are about three times more potent than bio-identical estrogens in stimulating the liver of a woman to produce renin, a substrate used to make angiotensin, which causes increased blood pressure.

None of the serious concerns raised by this research have been addressed by further studies in North America. It is also important to note that all of the studies indicating that estrogen replacement therapy leads to an increased risk of breast cancer were done using conjugated estrogens.

Despite information which would indicate bio-identical hormones are superior, synthetic conjugated estrogens remain the most frequently prescribed form of Estrogen Replacement Therapy (ERT). Metabolites of these synthetic estrogens have been linked to the development of breast cancer.

Structural differences in the estrogen molecules may account for some of the unpleasant side effects experienced by many women who take horse estrogens for HRT. In research and in clinical practice, natural bio-identical hormones have proven to be better tolerated and to have fewer side effects.

The early marketing of Premarin® was fueled by gynecologist Robert Wilson, M.D., in his book *Feminine Forever*, published in 1966. The book was written with the financial backing of the Ayerst laboratories. In his book, Wilson promoted menopause as a "deficiency disease", he campaigned to save women from the loss of their femininity. His view was that women were valued solely for their reproductive abilities and this "femininity" was what made them attractive to men. A direct quote from a paragraph in his book provides the general flavor of the book and the attitudes of many at the time...

> "The unpalatable truth must be faced that all postmenopausal women are castrates...from a practical point of view, a man remains a man until the very end. The situation with a woman is very different. Her ovaries become inadequate relatively early in life. She is the only mammal who cannot reproduce after middle age." *Feminine Forever* sold over 100,000 copies in seven months. The book was widely promoted in women's magazines with the effect that by 1975, there were approximately 6,000,000 women using Premarin® in this country alone.

Then, in 1975, in a report eerily similar to the latest NIH bombshell (see page 83), a study done at Kaiser-Permanente in San Francisco appeared in "The New England Journal of Medicine". The study showed that the women who took Premarin® were 7.6 times more at risk for endometrial cancer than those that didn't. Following this stunning revelation, Ayerst did not withdraw the product or go back to the drawing board for a better product, although they did reduce the recommended dosage. A new drug, Provera®, a synthetic progesterone, was added to the regimen to protect the uterus from endometrial cancer. The company began promoting Premarin/Provera® for the prevention of heart disease and osteoporosis. Here is where profit-motive began to overrun any semblance of science, as the campaign was initiated without the studies to support it. The company hired a public relations firm Burson-Marsteller, and paid doctors to travel around the country promoting their products for these conditions. The campaign hired writers to place stories in the national magazines to promote the great new benefits. Women were encouraged to take Premarin/Provera® for the rest of their lives. When the FCC lifted the ban on advertising drugs on television, Wyeth-Ayerst began using celebrities such as Lauren Hutton and Patti LaBelle in ads to promote their drugs. The campaign was remarkably successful. By the end of the 1990's, it was accepted, by almost all doctors who prescribed Premarin/Provera®, that the drugs provided protection against heart disease and osteoporosis.

Since then we have learned that all synthetic estrogen- and synthetic progesterone-like drugs (oral contraceptives, Premarin®, Tamoxifin®, Provera®, Prempro™, etc.) can cause cancer. There has been a dramatic rise in estrogen sensitive breast cancer. In fact, the majority of breast cancers in young women are estrogen sensitive caused by the greater exposure to estrogen and synthetic estrogen-like compounds.

Dr. Samuel Epstein's outstanding book, The Breast Cancer Prevention Program, outlines the role that synthetic estrogens play in causing breast cancer.

The lessons to be learned from these fiascos are:

1) Drug companies sell drugs.

2) Doctors prescribe drugs.
3) Doctors are influenced by drug companies and their own prejudices, not by scientific studies.
4) Doctors believe that nature made a mistake by allowing women to get pregnant.
5) Doctors believe that nature made a mistake by decreasing a woman's estrogen level, forcing them to go through menopause.
6) Doctors believe that most of life is a struggle against disease.

As prudent consumers we must courteously listen to our doctors. We must then question every one of their recommendations. Only then, after weighing the scientific evidence, should we proceed with any treatment plan.

Hippocrates, the father of modern medicine, said that the order of health is first - regimen, second - medicine and last - surgery. Regimen, according to Hippocrates consisted of lifestyle, diet, exercise, etc. Only after you exhaust regimen do you move onto medicine and only after you exhaust medicine do you move onto surgery. In this country we do things backwards. First we do surgery, if that fails we use medicine and if medicine fails we go to regimen. Following Hippocrates advice with regard to menopausal symptoms let us use regimen first, medicine secondarily and surgery only as a last resort.

We must remind the doctors of the oath of Hippocrates which they took upon graduating from medical school, "Primum Non Nocere" - Above All Do No

Harm. We must attempt to improve our life style with the following methods:

1) Avoid the birth control pill and hormone replacement therapy (synthetic altered estrogens and progesterones).
2) Avoid ingesting meat from animals that have been fed estrogen supplements and/or growth hormones.
3) Avoid milk from cows that have been injected with bovine growth hormone.

Nothing in life is a guarantee. Even if you follow the above principles, problems may still occur. However, statistically, you will lower your probability of problems. It is an upsetting thought that many of the diseases we will face in the 21st century will be caused by man, not nature produced.

Bottle feeding, vaccinations, synthetic hormones, and pesticides (such as DDT, dioxin, PCBs and PVCs) are just some of the factors which have been linked to the rise in cancer and auto immune diseases (Multiple Sclerosis, Hodgkins, Fibromyalgia, Chronic Fatigue Syndrome, etc.).

We are drowning in a sea of synthetic estrogens. Not only do our doctors use synthetic estrogens for acne, birth control, and then later in life for pre-menopause, and menopause, but we are also exposed to estrogen-like compounds in the form of xeno-estrogens (see pages 5, 128) and phyto-estrogens (see pages 3, 129). All of these synthetic estrogens have strongly contributed to the risks of endometrial cancer, breast cancer, and stroke. We have inadvertently created diseases as a result of synthetic estrogen overload. Other medications, like natural progesterone cream are required to overcome the effects of the excess estrogens to which we are exposed. Doctors finally realize that excess estrogen can lead to serious medical problems if not balanced by use of progcsterone. However, instead of adding natural progesterone, pharmaceutical companies create synthetic progesterones which not only do not effectively counteract the effects of estrogen, but cause their own set of serious problems.

Understanding the serious side effects of these synthetic estrogen and progesterone hormones is crucial to lowering the risk of cancer, heart disease, stroke, etc. You must control exposure to synthetic hormones, thereby reducing the incidence of these serious diseases.

The birth control pill is unavoidably dangerous; hormone replacement therapy is unavoidably dangerous. A majority of women in our society suffer from insufficient progesterone because of their high intake of estrogens and estrogen mimicking substances. The answer to these problems is not just adding additional progesterone, but involves the stopping of the intake of excess estrogen. If you are taking the birth control pill, stop. If you are taking synthetic hormone replacement therapy (Premarin®, Prempro™, etc.), find a doctor who will get you off these unavoidably dangerous medications. If the doctor prescribes the birth control pill for your teen age daughter for acne or to regulate her menstrual cycle, find another doctor. Life is not a disease that needs to be chemically balanced by synthetic products.

Scientific Literature Review

> *A survey of the scientific literature reveals that contrary to widely held physicians' beliefs, synthetic HRT does not protect against cardiac disease, stroke, gallbladder disease,* atherosclerosis *or diminished cognitive function.*

Synthetic Hormone Replacement Therapy and Heart Benefits

> ROCHESTER, Minnesota (MAYO CLINIC) - A new study raises questions about the cardiovascular benefits of estrogen-progestin hormone replacement therapy (HRT) in older women who already have heart disease.

A study of more than 2,700 middle-age and older women by Curt Furberg, M.D., of Wake Forest University, Winston-Salem, N.D., and colleagues found that daily use of an estrogen-progestin pill did not reduce the incidence of death or heart attack.

Dr. Furberg and colleagues found that those taking the estrogen-progestin pill actually had a higher risk of heart attacks and death during the first year than did those on the placebo, but had a lower risk during the final 2 years of the study.

The research raises questions about previous observational studies indicating that women on HRT have fewer heart attacks. The latest findings also raise questions about whether the apparent short-term risk of beginning hormone replacement therapy is offset by its potential long-term benefits.

"Based on the binding of no overall cardiovascular benefit and a pattern of early increase in risk of (coronary heart disease) events, we do not recommend starting this treatment for the purpose of secondary prevention of (coronary heart disease)," the authors conclude.

A cautionary note:

"There are two findings here that we should be cautious about," says Brooks S. Edwards, M.D., a cardiologist at Mayo Clinic, Rochester, Minn. "First, there seems to be an increase in cardiac events in the early period of hormone replacement therapy in women with coronary disease. Maybe the message here is, IF you have an unstable situation, maybe you shouldn't be introducing hormones at that time."

"Second, women in the study had an increase of venous thrombosis (blood clots) forming in the leg that sometimes traveled to the lung and caused damage," Dr. Edwards says. "Patients need to be aware of that risk too."

Hormone Therapy No Help For Heart Disease Prevention

WASHINGTON (Reuters) - August 18, 1998.

"I think that certainly women SHOULDN'T start taking it for the purpose of preventing heart disease because there's no proof that it works," Dr. Jacques Rossouw, who is conducting a similar, longer-term study at the National Heart, Lung and Blood Institute (NHLBI), said in a telephone interview.

ACC Report: Estrogen May Have Adverse Effects in Postmenopausal Women with CAD

NEW ORLEANS (Reuters Health) - March 11, 1999.

Duke investigators warned their colleagues here in attendance at the 48th annual meeting of the American College of Cardiology, that initiation of estrogen replacement therapy may actually increase the incidence of cardiac events in postmenopausal women with established coronary artery disease.

Dr. Karen P. Alexander presented data on more than 1,850 women with a history of myocardial infarction, who were enrolled in a 1996 study of the cardio-protective effects of aspirin. She reported that more than 37% of women who began hormone replacement therapy after study enrollment were hospitalized with unstable angina within one year.

In contrast, the hospitalization rate for women who had never used hormone replacement therapy was 17% and the rate for those already on hormone replacement therapy prior to aspirin therapy was 21%, Dr. Alexander told meeting participants.

The study results are similar to those reported last summer by a team at the University of California at San Francisco, Dr. Alexander said. In the earlier study, among women with heart disease who began estrogen replacement therapy after beginning either aspirin or coumadin to prevent reinfarction, nearly one third were hospitalized with unstable angina within a year. By comparison, the hospitalization rate was 21% in those already on estrogen prior to starting either aspirin or coumadin.

"While hormone use has benefits and may still be cardio-protective in women without heart disease, women who have heart disease should probably not start using [hormones]," Dr. Alexander said in a university statement. "We also have no reason to suggest women stop using hormones if they develop heart disease."

HRT AND PREVENTION OF CORONARY HEART DISEASE (CHD)

Excerpts from Dr. John Lee's Newsletter 1999

"...It is widely advertised that conventional HRT should be given to all postmenopausal women to prevent coronary heart disease. But is there good evidence for this claim? The reference most widely used to claim a heart benefit from HRT is the Nurses Questionnaire study, which was neither randomized, nor placebo controlled. A critique of this study appears in chapter 13 of Dr. Lee's book, "What Your Doctor May Not Tell You About Menopause" (see References). Recently JAMA published a randomized blinded study of 2,763 postmenopausal women followed for five years. One half of the women received Premarin® 0.625 mg and Provera® 2.5 mg. daily; and the other half received placebo. After five years of follow-up, there was no evidence of a cardiac benefit from hormone therapy. There was, however, a three-fold increase in the incidence of thromboembolic events [blood clots in the legs and lungs] and a significant increase in gallbladder disease in the treatment group compared to controls.

Similarly, the long-running Framingham study has compared the incidence of coronary heart disease with postmenopausal hormone replacement therapy and found no correlation."

If evidence-based medicine is your guide, the claim that HRT prevents CHD (coronary heart disease) must be discarded."

M.E. Comments:

Dr. John Lee was years ahead of his time with his recommendation that HRT should not be used for heart disease!

PHYSICIANS' COMMITTEE FOR RESPONSIBLE MEDICINE

ESTROGEN REPLACEMENT NOT ADVISABLE FOR OSTEOPOROSIS, HEART DISEASE

David Wasser, Media Director June 20, 1995

So why are so many doctors prescribing Hormone Replacement Therapy? Most of the push relates to osteoporosis and heart disease. Osteoporosis is very common in Caucasian women, less so among other races. About a quarter of white women over sixty have compression fractures of their vertebrae, and many develop hip fractures due to the gradual loss of bone. But estrogens are not nearly as good at protecting the bones as women may be led to believe, and they rarely arrest bone loss. At best, estrogens simply slow the rate of bone deterioration. Other approaches are much more effective, and they do not cause cancer. For example, a major article in the American Journal of Clinical Nutrition reported that eliminating meat from the diet can cut urinary calcium losses in half. This supports other studies showing that populations that follow plant-based diets have enviably low rates of hip fracture. Cutting salt intake can reduce calcium losses even further. Limiting caffeine consumption will hold onto still more calcium, and if patients don't smoke, they will avoid the 10% loss of bone that plagues chronic smokers.

For heart disease prevention, hormones are no match for lifestyle changes. But Americans want pills, and they don't want to be told to change their diets. According to PCRM, that's nonsense. It is patronizing to assume that every postmenopausal woman is too wedded to her current diet and lifestyle to listen to competent advice. The real problem is, she is not likely to find such advice. Most doctors know little about how diet affects health, even when a mountain of research has already been done, and is gathering dust in medical libraries. They rely instead on knee-jerk prescribing, which is continually encouraged by drug manufacturers' aggressive promotions. When doctors learn how to use all the tools their medical bags could really offer--including prescriptions for diet and lifestyle changes, their patients will be much better off.

Here are some interesting medical statistics:

Taking [synthetic] estrogen for 10 years increases the probability of developing breast cancer to about 10.7%; taking [synthetic] estrogen for 15 years may increase it to 13%, and has a 15% lifetime probability of having an osteoporotic hip fracture and a 1.5% probability of death from hip fracture. The median age of women for hip fracture is 79 years. This information is from "Menopause: Epidemiologic Aspects" by William R. Harlan, in Women's Health in Menopause, edited by P.G. Crosignani et al, Kluwer Academic Publishers, 1994.

In Annals of Internal Medicine, 3 July 2001 Volume 135 Number 1: 1-8, *"Postmenopausal Hormone Use and Secondary Prevention of Coronary Events in the Nurses' Health Study" A Prospective, Observational Study,* Meir J. Stampfer, M.D., et al., concluded that...

> ...In conclusion, results from HERS and the Nurses' Health Study, a large prospective, observational study, suggest that hormone therapy increases risk for a recurrent coronary event in the short term and that hormone therapy should not be initiated solely for prevention of recurrent heart disease.

ଓଓଃଓଓଃ

In Journal of American Medical Association, Vol. 288 No. 1, July 3, 2002, 49-57 *"Cardiovascular Disease Outcomes During 6.8 Years of Hormone Therapy" Heart and Estrogen/Progestin Replacement Study Follow-up (HERS II)* Deborah Grady, et al., found that...

> . . .The Heart and Estrogen/progestin Replacement Study (HERS) found no overall reduction in risk of coronary heart disease (CHD) events among postmenopausal women with CHD. However, in the hormone group, findings did suggest a higher risk of CHD events during the first year, and a decreased risk during years 3 to 5.

and concluded that

. . .Lower rates of CHD events among women in the hormone group in the final years of HERS did not persist during additional years of follow-up. After 6.8 years, hormone therapy did not reduce risk of cardiovascular events in women with CHD. Postmenopausal hormone therapy should not be used to reduce risk for CHD events in women with CHD.

. . .**Financial Disclosures:** During the conduct of HERS, all authors were supported by contracts from Wyeth-Ayerst. Dr Grady received research support from Berlex and Eli Lilly. Dr Herrington receives research support from Eli Lilly and Parke-Davis/Pfizer, and occasional honoraria from Wyeth-Ayerst and Eli Lilly. Dr Bittner has grants from Wyeth-Ayerst (ancillary study to HERS), Pfizer, and Merck (both cholesterol studies); and is also on the speaker's bureau for Pfizer and Merck and has attended a consultant meeting for Merck-Schering Plough. Dr Blumenthal has received clinical research support and honoraria to speak at educational conferences from the following companies that make lipid lowering drugs and/or anti-hypertensive drugs: Merck, Pfizer, Kos Pharmaceuticals, and Bristol-Myers Squibb. Dr Wenger's potential conflicts of interest are Eli Lilly Raloxifene Advisory Committee, Heart

Disease in Women, MED-ED, Pfizer Inc, Coalition for the Advancement of Cardiovascular Health, Cardiology Consultants, Pfizer Inc.

Funding/Support: This study was funded by Wyeth-Ayerst Research.

Role of the Sponsor: Wyeth-Ayerst Research funded the study, contributed to its design, oversaw quality control at the clinical centers including periodic site visits, and edited the data collected by the clinical centers (except for disease outcome data) before sending it to the coordinating center at University of California, San Francisco. The sponsor did not have access to the blinding code, and played no role in collecting or adjudicating disease outcomes nor in data analysis. **The sponsor had the opportunity to review and comment on manuscripts that had been written by the investigators, but our contract gave the investigators the final decision as to content.**

M.E. Comments:

This major study in JAMA, funded in large part by Wyeth-Ayerst Research, adds more evidence that synthetic estrogen and progestin not only do not protect against heart disease, but may actually contribute to it. Wyeth must have been so sure of the outcome before the study that contrary to their typical contracts, which allow them the right to refuse to have the study published in the event that the outcome is unfavorable to them, they left the final decision to the investigators, a clear benefit to the public. I hope doctors will now stop prescribing synthetic HRT for prevention of cardiovascular disease. However, if your doctor still recommends synthetic HRT, and tells you that it will help your heart, my recommendation is to find another doctor.

Synthetic Hormone Replacement Therapy and Stroke

In the *New England Journal of Medicine* Volume 345:1243-1249 October 25, 2001 Number 17, Catherine M. Viscoli, et al., studied "A Clinical Trial of Estrogen-Replacement Therapy after Ischemic Stroke" and found that...

> Observational studies have suggested that estrogen-replacement therapy may reduce a woman's risk of stroke and death and found that during a mean follow-up period of 2.8 years, there were 99 strokes or deaths among the women in the estradiol group, and 93 among those in the placebo group (relative risk in the estradiol group, 1.1; 95 percent confidence interval, 0.8 to 1.4). . .
>
> ... In this high-risk population of postmenopausal women with a recent cerebrovascular event, treatment with estradiol-17 for three years was ineffec-

tive in reducing the overall risk of stroke or death or the incidence of the individual end points of death, fatal or nonfatal stroke, transient ischemic attack, or cardiac events during follow-up. Moreover, this therapy was associated with adverse effects on the endometrium, including elevated rates of vaginal bleeding and endometrial hyperplasia and a more frequent need for hysterectomy.

Although we cannot rule out the possibility that estrogen therapy has minimal cerebrovascular benefits, our study had sufficient power to rule out reductions in the risk of death or stroke of more than 20 percent. . .

... The ongoing Women's Health Initiative, a randomized trial, should help clarify the role of estrogen in the primary prevention of cardiovascular disease, including stroke. Our results indicate that estrogen therapy should not be initiated for the purpose of secondary prevention of cerebrovascular disease and add to the evolving body of evidence from clinical trials that do not show a benefit of estrogen for women with established vascular disease.

And concluded that . . .

Estradiol does not reduce mortality or the recurrence of stroke in

postmenopausal women with cerebrovascular disease. This therapy should not be prescribed for the secondary prevention of cerebrovascular disease.

Supported by a grant (1-RO1-N531251) from the National Institute of Neurological Disorders and Stroke and by Mead Johnson Laboratories, which also provided the study drug. Dr. Suissa was supported by a Senior Scientist Award from the Medical Research Council of Canada.

Drs. Viscoli, Brass, Kernan, Suissa, and Horwitz have received research support from Novartis. Dr. Suissa has also received research funding from Schering and Organon.

***M.E. Comments*:**

Vicoli, et al's study adds to the growing body of evidence that HRT does not reduce the risk of mortality or recurrence of stroke in post-menopausal women with cerebrovascular disease. In fact one year later, the Women's Health Initiative Study will show that it actually increases cerebral vascular mortality and morbidity.

Synthetic Hormone Replacement Therapy and Breast Cancer

In the *Journal of the American Medical Association,* Vol. 283 No. 4, January 26, 2000 :485-491"Menopausal Estrogen and Estrogen-Progestin Replacement Therapy and Breast Cancer Risk" Catherine Schairer, et al., studied

> Whether menopausal hormone replacement therapy using a combined estrogen-progestin regimen increases risk of breast cancer beyond that associated with estrogen alone is unknown.

and concluded that . . .

> Our data suggest that the estrogen-progestin regimen increases breast cancer risk beyond that associated with estrogen alone.

Synthetic Hormone Replacement Therapy and Ovarian Cancer

NATIONAL CANCER INSTITUTE News from the NCI

Office of Communications/ Mass Media Branch/
Building 31, Room 10A19, Bethesda, MD 20892
National Institutes of Health : NCI Press Office (301) 496-6641

EMBARGOED FOR RELEASE
4:00 p.m. EDT
July 16, 2002

Definitions of Scientific Terms

Increased Risk of Ovarian Cancer is Linked to Estrogen Replacement Therapy

Researchers from the National Cancer Institute (NCI) have found that women in a large study who used estrogen replacement therapy after menopause were at increased risk for ovarian cancer. The report was published in the July 17, 2002, issue of *JAMA.**

The scientists followed 44,241 women for approximately 20 years. Compared to postmenopausal women not using hormone replacement therapy, users of estrogen-only therapy had a 60 percent greater risk of developing ovarian cancer. The risk increased with length of estrogen use. The women, who were followed from 1979 to 1998, were former participants in the Breast Cancer Detection Demonstration Project, a mammography screening program conducted between 1973 and 1980.

"The main finding of our study was that postmenopausal women who used estrogen replacement therapy for 10 or more years were at significantly higher risk of developing ovarian cancer than women who never used hormone replacement therapy," said James V. Lacey, Jr., Ph.D., lead author of the study from NCI's Division of Cancer Epidemiology and Genetics. The relative risk for 10 to 19 years of use was 1.8, which translates to an 80 percent higher risk than non-users, and increased to 3.2 (a 220 percent higher risk than non-users) for women who took estrogen for 20 or more years.

Estrogen is a natural hormone produced primarily by the ovaries. After menopause, the ovaries produce lower levels of the hormones estrogen and progesterone. By the time natural menopause is complete - usually between ages 45 and 55 - hormone output decreases significantly. As early as the 1940s, women began using estrogens in high doses to counteract some of the short-term discomforts of menopause (hot flashes, vaginal drying and thinning, and urinary tract incontinence and infections).

However, after it became clear in the 1970s that women who took estrogen alone had a six to eight times higher risk of developing endometrial cancer (cancer of the lining of the uterus), doctors began prescribing progestin along with much lower doses of estrogen. Progestin is a synthetic form of the natural hormone progesterone. The addition of progestin to estrogen therapy reduces the increased risk of endometrial cancer associated with using estrogen alone. As a result, it has become increasingly common to prescribe estrogen-progestin therapy for women who have not had a hysterectomy.

In addition to studying the effect of estrogen use alone, Lacey and his colleagues looked at whether women using estrogen-progestin therapy were more likely to develop ovarian cancer. No increased risk was found.

Lacey commented, "Even though our data showed that women who took estrogen combined with progestin were not at increased risk for ovarian cancer, only a few women in our study who developed ovarian cancer had used estrogen-progestin therapy for more than four years. So, at this point, there simply aren't enough data to say whether taking the combined therapy has any effect on ovarian cancer."

Past studies suggested that postmenopausal hormone treatments might be effective in preventing or reducing some of the negative long-term effects of aging, such as heart disease and osteoporosis. However, the results from a large multi-center clinical trial, also published in the July 17 issue of *JAMA* (*JAMA* 2002;288:321-333), showed increases in breast cancer, coronary heart disease, stroke, and blood clots in the lungs and legs for women on estrogen-progestin therapy for an average of 5.2 years. The trial, part of the Women's Health Initiative (WHI),0 also found fewer cases of hip fractures and colon cancer among women taking the combined therapy. However, because overall the harm was greater than the benefit, the trial was stopped last week, three years ahead of schedule. The WHI randomized trial for estrogen alone in women who have had their uterus removed is continuing.

Lacey emphasized the complexity of weighing the various risks and benefits of hormone use. "Because hormone therapy may influence so many conditions that affect women after menopause - cardiovascular disease, osteoporosis, breast cancer, uterine cancer, gallbladder disease, blood clots, and now potentially ovarian cancer - we should no longer think of a woman basing her decision to use hormones on the potential risk of just one condition. Women should continue to talk to their health care providers about whether hormones might be right for them."

Previous studies looking at the effect of postmenopausal hormones on ovarian cancer risk have been inconsistent. Some reported increased risk with estrogen use while others reported either no effect or a protective one. Most of these earlier studies were relatively small and limited by incomplete information about ovarian cancer risk factors.

Two recent large studies found a link between hormone use and ovarian cancer. A large prospective study published last year (*JAMA* 2001;285:1460-1465) showed that postmenopausal estrogen use for 10 or more years was associated with increased risk of ovarian cancer mortality, and a recent Swedish study (*J. Natl. Cancer Inst.* 2002;94:497-504) reported that estrogen use alone and estrogen-progestin used sequentially (progestin used on average 10 days/month) may be associated with an increased risk for ovarian cancer. In contrast, estrogen-progestin used continuously (progestin used on average 28 days/month) seemed to confer no increased ovarian cancer risk.

Lacey said that some of the unknowns concerning hormone use and ovarian cancer include the following:

• • Duration vs. dose of estrogen therapy
It is not clear from this study whether the increased risk with estrogen use is due to higher doses of estrogen, longer duration of estrogen use, or both dose and duration. It is also not clear whether long-term use of lower-dose estrogen is associated with ovarian cancer.

• • Duration of estrogen-progestin therapy
Most women in this study were on the combined therapy for less than four years, so more data will be needed to determine whether estrogen-progestin use increases risk. The effect of long-term use of estrogen-progestin therapy is not known.

• • The type of estrogen-progestin regimen
The continuous regimen involves taking both hormones simultaneously throughout the month. The sequential regimen, on the other hand, involves taking estrogen every day, and progestin for 10 to 14 days each month.

• • Use of more than one type of hormone replacement therapy
For instance, after taking estrogen alone, some women changed to a combined regimen after reports of increased endometrial cancer risk with estrogen alone. More data are needed to analyze the effect of switching from one regimen to another.

• • The form of estrogen administration
Most studies have analyzed the use of estrogens in pill form, but it can also be administered by patches, shots, and creams.

Every year, about 23,000 U.S. women are diagnosed with ovarian cancer and 14,000 women die from the disease. A woman's lifetime risk of developing ovarian cancer is 1.7 percent. This means that in a group of 100 women followed from birth to age 85, fewer than two would get ovarian cancer. In comparison, about 13 women would get breast cancer (lifetime risk is 13.3 percent), fewer than three women would develop uterine cancer (lifetime risk is 2.7 percent), and between 16 and 32 women would develop osteoporosis.

An estimated 40 million U.S. women will experience menopause during the next 20 years, and women today are living approximately one-third of their life after menopause.

Anywhere from 20 percent to 45 percent of U.S. women take some form of hormone therapy between the ages of 50 and 75. According to industry estimates, about 8 million U.S. women use estrogen alone and about 6 million U.S. women use estrogen-progestin therapy. About 20 percent of hormone users continue for more than five years.

* "Menopausal hormone replacement therapy and risk of ovarian cancer." The authors are James V. Lacey, Jr., Pamela J. Mink, Jay H. Lubin, Mark E. Sherman, Rebecca Troisi, Patricia Hartge, Arthur Schatzkin, and Catherine Schairer. *JAMA* 2002;288:334-341.

SYNTHETIC HORMONE REPLACEMENT THERAPY AND GALLBLADDER DISEASE

In Annals of Internal Medicine, 2 October 2001 Volume 135 Number 7: 493-501, *"Effect of Estrogen plus Progestin on Risk for Biliary Tract Surgery in Postmenopausal Women with Coronary Artery Disease" The Heart and Estrogen/progestin Replacement Study*, Joel A. Simon, MD, MPH; Donald B. Hunninghake, MD; Sanjay K. Agarwal, MD; Feng Lin, MS; Jane A. Cauley, DrPH; Christine C. Ireland, MPH; James H. Pickar, MD, for the Heart and Estrogen/progestin Replacement Study (HERS) Research Group studied the effect of taking . . .

> Conjugated equine estrogens, 0.625 mg, plus medroxyprogesterone acetate, 2.5 mg, daily in one tablet or identical placebo.

And found that. . .

> Data from the Third National Health and Nutrition Examination Survey indicate that 11% of U.S. women have a history of clinical gallbladder disease——that is, either previous cholecystectomy or self-reported history of gallstones. Factors associated with gallbladder disease, at least in some studies, include older age, female sex, white ethnicity/race, obesity, rapid weight loss, and, among women, greater parity, use of oral estrogen––containing contraceptives, and postmenopausal estrogen therapy . These associations, in

general, have been based on observational data and may partly reflect the effects of ascertainment and recall bias, as well as confounding. While some observational studies suggest that estrogens increase the risk for gallbladder disease by as much as twofold to fourfold, such an association has not been reported consistently. The effect of combined estrogen plus progestin therapy has been less well studied, and no recent clinical trial data exist on the relation of such therapy to the risk for biliary tract surgery among postmenopausal women.

To determine whether estrogen plus progestin therapy is associated with the risk for biliary tract surgery among postmenopausal women, we analyzed data from the Heart and Estrogen/progestin Replacement Study (HERS), the first large randomized, double-blind trial of estrogen plus progestin therapy for the secondary prevention of coronary heart disease. Gallbladder disease events, including biliary tract surgery, were among several prespecified secondary outcomes of interest.

With results that...

Gallbladder disease was particularly prevalent among this cohort of postmenopausal women with coronary artery

> disease. Twenty-three percent of women reported a history of cholelithiasis or cholecystectomy at baseline
>
> ...the HERS cohort included older women with coronary disease, among whom clinical gallbladder disease was highly prevalent at baseline. For these reasons, our findings may not be generalizable to other populations of women. However, to our knowledge, our study is the only large, randomized, double-blind trial of estrogen plus progestin therapy to examine the effect of such therapy on the risk for biliary tract surgery, and our findings are unlikely to reflect confounding or bias.

And concluded that...

> postmenopausal hormone therapy tended to increase the risk for biliary tract surgery among women in HERS, who had coronary artery disease and were followed for an average of 4.1 years.

Role of the Funding Source

> Wyeth-Ayerst Research funded HERS. The study was designed and carried out by the HERS investigators, including scientists from Wyeth-Ayerst Research. Investigators at the HERS Coordinating Center at the University of California, San Francisco, collected the outcome data,

supervised the adjudication of outcome events, and analyzed the data.

Synthetic Hormone Replacement Therapy and Cognitive Function

In *American Journal Epidemiology* 2001; 154:733-739, "Estrogen replacement therapy may not prevent decline in cognitive functioning" Suzana Alves de Moraes et al., concluded:

> ...Despite encouraging findings from animal studies, estrogen replacement therapy appears not to retard a decline in cognitive functioning in postmenopausal women.

ƆƷƆƷ

Synthetic Hormone Replacement Therapy and Atherosclerosis

In *American Journal Epidemiology* 2002; 156:438-444, [Synthetic] "HRT does not prevent atherosclerosis after oophorectomy" Kathleen M. Dwyer, et al., found...

> **Endogenous hormones, but not synthetic (see page 3) hormone replacement therapy (HRT) are protective against the development of subclinical atherosclerosis.**

References

Berger, Gary S., M.D., The Couples' Guide to Infertility, 1995.

Couple to Couple League's website is http://www.ccli.org

Epstein, Steinman, LeVert, The Breast Cancer Prevention Program,"Chapter 3, The Pill: Assessing Your Risks." Macmillan, U.S.A.

http://www.homefirst.com (The Homefirst® WEB page containing extensive links to research on "the Pill", as well as many related topics).

Lee, M.D., John R., What Your Doctor May *Not* Tell You about PREMENOPAUSE, (Balancing Your Hormones and Your Life From Thirty to Fifty) Warner Books, 1999.

Women considering synthetic hormone replacement therapy (HRT) for menopause symptoms and health benefits should read this book first. Lee has studied the research and concludes that estrogen is not the magic bullet for protection against heart disease and osteoporosis, nor does it retard aging. Natural progesterone, instead, puts postmenopausal women's hormones in balance. Dr. Lee cites study after study that indicates that natural progesterone, obtained in cream form, delivers what the synthetic HRT only promises.

Lee, M.D., John. What Your Doctor May Not Tell You About Menopause: The Breakthrough Book on Natural Progesterone, 1996.

Lee, M.D., John. What Your Doctor May Not Tell You About Breast Cancer 2002.

Martin, Gerstung. The Estrogen Alternative: Natural Hormone Therapy With Botanical Progesterone, Healing Arts Press, 1998.

Mintz, Morton The Pill An Alarming Report, (*Washington Post)* 1969.

Ratner, Herbert, M.D., The Medical Hazards of the Birth Control Pill, "Child and Family" 1970.

Seaman, Barbara, The Doctor's Case Against the Pill, 1995 (original publication 1969), Hunter House.

Theo Colborn, et al, Our Stolen Future, Penguin Group, 1997.

Wright, Jonathan, V., M.D., Natural Hormone Replacement For Women Over 45; Smart Publications, 1997.

CHAPTER II

ESTROGEN - THE COMMON LINK TO BREAST CANCER

Estrogen is intimately connected with the development of most breast cancers. Estrogen encourages breast cells to divide more often and more rapidly. Thus, if a mutation (inherited or triggered by a carcinogen) lies imbedded in the DNA, cancer cells are more likely to proliferate when high estrogen levels are present. This also may help to explain why breast cancer rates in women have increased in tandem with the widespread use of Hormone Replacement Therapy and Birth Control Pills. Both of these synthetic hormonal medications increase the amount of estrogen circulating in a woman's body. Indeed, we now know that two distinct types of breast cancer exist: the far more common, estrogen-dependent breast cancer influenced primarily by estrogen, and the less common, non-estrogen dependent breast cancer. More than 75% of women with breast cancer have estrogen-dependent cancers, and that number is increasing at a particularly alarming rate. According to a study published in 1990 by the Journal of the National Cancer Institute, the incidence of estrogen-dependent breast cancers, particularly among post-menopausal women, increased by 130% from mid-1970's to the mid-1980's in contrast to only a 27% increase in non-estrogen-dependent cancers. A 1997 study in the same journal confirmed these findings.

Contrary to what you may have heard or read, synthetic Hormone Replacement Therapy and oral contraceptives ("the Pill"), do not protect against heart disease. They do cause increased blood clots, cancer, strokes, etc. and there are other safer means to prevent osteoporosis. Estrogen replacement therapy is an avoidable cause of breast cancer. Risks are greatest with prolonged use and high doses and also with estrogen-progestin combinations.

The birth control pills: first, second and third generations are avoidably dangerous drugs. With every subsequent generation of birth control pills the dangers did not decline. Birth control pills are contraindicated especially for women with benign breast disease, with a family history of breast cancer, or who began taking oral contraceptives in their teen years, especially before a first full term pregnancy (FFTP) (see page 148).

Doctors and the public have been indoctrinated as to the medicinal value of HRT and the birth control pill. Doctors believe that pregnancy is a disease to be avoided and that menopause is a fate worse than death. They use that belief as a reason to dose a woman with estrogen from her reproductive years through menopause. Doctors continue to ignore the growing body of evidence as to the risks of synthetic hormone use. Even when the evidence demonstrates a very strong association between synthetic estrogens and breast and endometrial cancers, doctors refuse to change their position (see page 122). They argue that synthetic estrogens are still valuable because they truly believe that new studies will show that synthetic HRT is not that dangerous.

There is no benefit in taking synthetic estrogens to prevent heart disease. The benefits that synthetic hormones allegedly have in preventing osteoporosis are not only questionable, but the same or better results can be obtained by diet, exercise and the application of the safe, natural progesterone creams.

A Survey of the Scientific Literature Estrogen, Abortion and Cancer

National Right to Life News - August 12, 1997

> Estradiol (one of the bodies natural estrogens) increases 20 times higher during the first trimester of pregnancy. If the pregnancy is completed the growth of breast tissue is halted and replaced with milk producing tissues. Thus, if pregnancy is stopped short by abortion, or breast feeding is not used, the excess estrogen level in blood may promote breast tissue to grow abnormally into cancerous cells.
>
> Pregnancies which terminate spontaneously or naturally are associated with low estrogen levels and thus do not present the problem of excess estrogen stimulation.

Birth Control Pills (Synthetic Estrogen Hormones)

http:/www.web.tusco.net/newone/estrogen.htm

Birth control pills usually contain about .1 mg. of synthetic estrogen and about 2 mg. of synthetic progesterone. The administration of birth control pills prevents the female body from producing the natural hormones resulting in no egg formation or not further development of a fertilized egg (a chemically induced abortion). Natural estrogen and natural progesterone metabolize or oxidize quickly and there to be effective as contraceptives they have to be administered via injection or trans-dermally. Synthetic analogs, which have slightly different chemical structures, do not metabolize or oxidize quickly and thus could be used in pill form. Unfortunately, the synthetic hormones can accumulate in the human body in very high dosages. The level of natural estrogen in the adult body is about 2 to 20 ppt (parts per trillion). The .1 mg. found in birth control pills amounts to about 300,000 ppt for a woman who weighs 160 pounds. Doses of xeno-estrogen (such as DDT, PCBs which act like human estrogen) chemicals at 2,000 parts ppt are already enough to produce abnormality in the reproductive system of clinical rats. RU 486, the abortion inducing chemical, is a synthetic analog of natural progesterone. It has similar chemical structure to natural progesterone but functions much differently. Progesterone is the key hormone in the adult female body which establishes and maintains normal pregnancy. RU486, due to the similar structure, will trick the body to accept it instead of progesterone and due to its high dose the body will stop secreting the natural progesterone hormone which is vital in nurturing the embryo which consequently will die in the uterus. RU486 is recommended to be used for 2 days and 600 mg. level which equals to 10,000,000 ppt or about 1,000,000 times a higher concentration than the normal level in the adult female body.

Estrogen and Breast Cancer

New England Journal of Medicine 2/27/97... CNN Internet, "New Study Links Estrogen Treatment and Breast Cancer"...

When researchers tracked 1300 women for 25 years, they found that those who had the most dense bones were 3.5 times more likely to develop breast cancer than those with the least dense bones. The researchers say a woman's bone mass may be a way of measuring her estrogen exposure over time. Knowing her estrogen exposure may help to predict her risk of breast cancer... The researchers also say it may be a woman's lifetime exposure to estrogen that would increase her chances of developing breast cancer – not necessarily estrogen taken during and after menopause."

THE HARVARD NURSES HEALTH STUDY - JULY 1997

The recent update from the *Harvard Nurses Health Study* has linked the long-term effects of HRT with breast cancer. The Harvard study which followed 121,700 nurses found that HRT for five or more years after menopause increased a woman's breast cancer risk by 30% if she takes estrogen alone and 40% if she's on estrogen and progestin

"MENOPAUSE" - 1998 FALL; 5(3): 145-51, BRINTON, LA

Breast cancer risk among women under 55 years of age by joint effects of usage of oral contraceptives and hormone replacement therapy.

A case control study of breast cancer among women under the age of 55 years in was held in Atlanta, Georgia.

> Results: Use of oral contraceptives was associated with a relative risk of 1.1 whereas the relative risk for hormone replacement therapy was .9. When the combined effects of longer use of both agents were considered, subjects who reported use of oral contraceptives for 10 or more years and hormone replacement for 3 or more years had a relative risk of 3.2 compared with non-users of either preparation. (A relative risk of 3.2 means it is 320 times more likely than the non-user population.)

and concluded...

> This study raises the necessity of further evaluation of breast cancer risk from the increase in the common exposure to both oral contraceptives and hormone replacement therapy.

HRT Link to Breast Cancer Risk

In the *Journal of the National Cancer Institute*, 1998; 90:814-823, Dr. Graham Colditz of Harvard Medical School in Boston, Massachusetts wrote...

> Hormone replacement therapy appears to increase the risk of breast cancer in post-menopausal women,

> according to a review of available data published in the "Journal of the American Cancer Institute". An analysis of 51 studies involving more than 150,000 women with and without breast cancer found that each year of hormone use increased the risk of breast cancer by 2.3%.

In the *Journal National Cancer Institute* 1998;90:1292-1299, "High Level of Estrogen Increases Breast Cancer Risk for Postmenopausal Women" Dr. Susan E. Hankinson, of Harvard Medical School, Boston, Mass found that...

> "A high plasma level of estrogen is associated with an increased risk of breast cancer among postmenopausal women, according to the results of a case controlled study conducted as part of the nurses health study."

In the *Annals Internal Medicine* 1999;130:262-269. "Hormone Replacement Therapy Linked to Increase in Breast Tissue Density" Dr. Elizabeth Barrett-Connor, of the University of California San Diego found...

> "Hormone replacement therapy, particularly estrogen-progestin regiments, significantly increases mammographic density in the first year of use, potentially increasing the risk of breast cancer."

In *Endocrinology and Metabolism Clinics* Vol. 26, No. 2, June 1997, "Hormone Replacement Therapy and Risk for Breast Cancer" Louis A. Brinton, Ph.D., Environmental Epidemiology Branch, National Cancer Institute found that...

> An influence of estrogens on breast cancer was acknowledged as early as 1886 when a palliative effect of oophorectomy on advanced breast cancer was described... Menopausal estrogens have become one of the most widely used drugs. An estimated 31.7 million prescriptions for oral medications were dispensed in 1992."

In *JAMA* Vol. 283 No. 4, January 2000, "Menopausal Estrogen and Estrogen-Progestin Replacement Therapy and Breast Cancer Risk"Schairer, Catherine, et al. found that...

> Using estrogen combined with progesterone for hormone replacement therapy (HRT) for more than a few years increases a woman's risk of breast cancer far beyond that she would experience without the therapy [HRT]...
>
> ...Compared with women who received no hormone therapy, women who took estrogen and progesterone in combination for an average of 3.5 years had a 40% greater chance of developing

> breast cancer. The risks were also calculated based on each subsequent year of use. Women on estrogen alone had an increased risk of 1% a year for each year of use, compared with the women on the estrogen-progesterone combination, for whom the increase was 8% a year. [Editor's note: the estrogen in all of these studies is synthetic, not natural estrogen and the progesterone, is not natural progesterone it is a synthetic progestin].

ଓଃଓଃ

In Estrogen & Breast Cancer - A Warning to Women, Hunter House, 1996:170-171, Rinzler, CarolAnn writes that...

> ...throughout the 1980's as the incidence of breast cancer in the United States continued to rise, American women and their doctors searched for a reasonable explanation for the epidemic... The explanation is this: Exposure to estrogen-both the estrogen produced in a woman's body and the [synthetic] estrogen she takes in a variety of drugs - increases the risk of breast cancer... In the end we must accept the evidence before our eyes without fear or prejudice. It is our only hope for defeating this disease.

***M.E. Comments**:*
*The scientific evidence is overwhelming as to the link between estrogen and breast cancer. Hormones only work if the receptor site is present on the cell. Tests have been developed to determine whether or not breast cancer cells have receptors for estrogen and progesterone. If the cancer cells are **estrogen** receptor (page 2) positive, estrogen must be avoided because estrogen causes the cancer cells to multiply. If the cancer cells are **progesterone** receptor (page 4) positive, it means the cells are receptive to the effects of progesterone. The theory is that progesterone may counteract the estrogen and inhibit the growth of the cancer cells. Progesterone is the antagonist to estrogen. It may very well be that giving progesterone to a woman with breast cancer who is both estrogen and progesterone receptor positive may inhibit the growth of the cancer cells. More research is needed to confirm the balancing effect of progesterone on the cancer cells.*

References

Berger, Gary S. Dr. ,The Couples' Guide to Infertility, 1995.

Couple to Couple League's website is http://www.ccli.org

Epstein, Steinman, LeVert, The Breast Cancer Prevention Program, - "Chapter 3, The Pill: Assessing Your Risks" Macmillan, U.S.A.

Lee, John M.D., What Your Doctor May Not Tell You About Menopause: The Breakthrough Book on Natural Progesterone, 1996.

Lee, M.D., John R., What Your Doctor May *Not* Tell You about PREMENOPAUSE, (Balancing Your Hormones and Your Life From Thirty to Fifty) Warner Books, 1999.

Women considering synthetic hormone replacement therapy (HRT) for menopause symptoms and health benefits should read this book first. Lee has studied the research and concludes that estrogen is not the magic bullet for protection against heart disease and osteoporosis, nor does it retard aging. Natural progesterone, instead, puts postmenopausal women's hormones in balance. Dr. Lee cites study after study which indicate that natural progesterone, obtained in cream form, delivers what the synthetic HRT only promises.

Martin, Gerstung, The Estrogen Alternative: Natural Hormone Therapy With Botanical Progesterone, Healing Arts Press, 1998.

Mintz, Morton "The Pill An Alarming Report," Washington Post 1969.

Ratner, Herbert M.D., "The Medical Hazards of the Birth Control Pill," Child and Family 1970.

Rinzler, CarolAnn, Estrogen & Breast Cancer - A Warning to Women, Hunter House, 1996.

Why breast cancer has reached epidemic proportions. How HRT and the Pill have contributed to its rise. What women and their doctors can do to reduce the risks.

Schairer, Catherine, et al, *JAMA* Vol. 283 No. 4, 2000 "Menopausal Estrogen and Estrogen-Progestin Replacement Therapy and Breast Cancer Risk"

Seaman, Barbara The Doctor's Case Against the Pill, 1995 (original publication 1969), Hunter House.

Wright, M.D., Jonathan, V. Natural Hormone Replacement For Women Over 45; Smart Publications, 1997.

www.homefirst.com (The Homefirst® WEB page containing extensive links to research on HRT, Oral Contraceptives, Natural Progesterone Cream and synthetic hormone replacement therapy, as well as many related topics).

CHAPTER III

SYNTHETIC ESTROGEN AND THE NATIONAL TOXICOLOGY PROGRAM

Every two years the National Toxicology Program (NTP) a Division of the U.S. Department of Health and Human Services (HHS) publishes a list of carcinogens, and recommends that they be included in the RoC (Report on Carcinogens).

> ...The evaluation of substances listed in the Report is performed by scientists from the National Toxicology Program, other Federal health research and regulatory agencies, and non government institutions.

...For the purpose of this Report,

> ***known to be human carcinogens*** are defined as those substances for which there is sufficient evidence of carcinogenicity from human studies that indicates a causal relationship between exposure to the agent, substance, mixture or exposure circum-stance and human cancer. Human studies are defined as human epidemiology studies and/or experimental studies of human tissues or cells. These experimental studies could include metabolic and toxicokinetic considerations as well as evidence of genetic damage, DNA binding, or

persistence of DNA lesions in exposed humans.

Reasonably anticipated to be human carcinogens are those substances for which there is limited evidence of carcinogenicity in humans and/or sufficient evidence of carcinogenicity in experimental animals. Sufficient evidence in animals is demonstrated by positive carcinogenicity findings in multiple species, or at multiple tissue sites, or by multiple routes of exposure, or to an unusual degree with regard to incidence, site or type of tumor or age at onset. There may be substances for which there is less than sufficient evidence of carcinogenicity in humans or laboratory animals but for which there are compelling data indicating that the substance could cause cancer in humans. Conversely, there may be substances for which there is evidence of carcinogenicity in laboratory animals but there are compelling data indicating that the agent acts through mechanisms which do not operate in humans and would therefore not reasonably be anticipated to cause cancer in humans. Conclusions regarding carcinogenicity in humans or experimental animals are based on scientific judgment, with consideration given to all relevant information. Relevant information includes, but is not limited to dose response, route of exposure, chemical structure, metabolism, pharmacokinetics, sensitive sub populations, genetic effects or other data relating to mechanism of action, and/or factors that may be unique to a given substance or exposure circumstance.

In December 2000 the National Toxicology Program recommended that steriodal estrogens (see page 5), which are widely used in menopausal therapy and in oral contraceptives for women, be listed in the "10th Report on Carcinogens" (RoC) as **"known to be human carcinogens"**.

After the Committee recommends a substance be placed in the RoC as a "known to be human carcinogen," federal law requires that the public be asked to comment. Following are some of the comments, by public citizens with regard to steriodal estrogens.

Public Comments Submitted to the 10th Report on Carcinogens With Reference to Adding Steriodal Estrogens to the list of "Known to be Human Carcinogens"

February 19, 2001

Dr. C.W. Jameson
National Toxicology Program
Report on Carcinogens
P.O. Box 12233
79 Alexander Dr. Bld. 4401 Rm. 3127
Research Triangle Park, NC 27709

Dear Dr. Jameson,

I am a 27 year-old breast cancer patient, desperately urging your panel to follow through with the recommendation made back in December to include sterodial estrogens in the 10th Report on Carcinogens. I was diagnosed in August 2000. I have no family history of breast cancer (or *any* other cancer) on either side of my family, traceable back five generations. I have also tested negative for the BRCA 1&2 gene mutations. I do not drink alcohol and I do not smoke (and never did). I am thin, and I always ate healthily and exercised regularly.

My only apparent risk factor was my use of **oral contraceptives for 10 years** from ages 17- 27. I did not know that this was a risk factor for breast cancer. I was never told this by **ANY** medical provider (**until *after* my diagnosis!**). There was no mention of the possibility of breast cancer in my pill package insert "**warning**" label.

Through my own research, I have found over 15 medical studies confirming the link between early onset of breast cancer and early and prolonged oral contraceptive use. One particularly notable study was a 1994 NCI study demonstrating an increased risk of *70%* of developing breast cancer before age 35 for women who used the pill before age 20 and who took it for at least 5 years. Additionally I have met several other brave young women who like me, are breast cancer victims who used oral contraceptives containing sterodial estrogens for many years. Incidentally, breast cancer rates for younger women are rising; considering that approximately 11 million American women use oral contraceptives- this could be one of the reasons.

I never knew that I was ingesting a known human carcinogen every day for 10 years, and if I had known, I would not have used that method of contraception.
My particular brand of pill, (Nordette: manufactured by Wyeth-Averst) contained ethinyl estradiol. I am confident that my use of sterodial estrogens for 10 years played a significant role in the development of (and most likely caused) my cancer.
I am certainly not alone in this thinking, the data supports my theory. Women deserve to be warned of this preventable risk, please remember me (and the other approx. 182,000 women who will be diagnosed with breast cancer in 2001) to put a face on those statistics; the use of sterodial estrogens is NOT an acceptable risk.

Please accept this letter as part of the "public comment" which the NTP solicited regarding the potential placement of sterodial estrogens on the report. Thank you for your consideration.

Sincerely,

Monica Bellenger

MONICA BELLENGER
1506 S. Barrington Ave. #203
Los Angels, CA 90025
(310) 268-0209

ANNE S. KASPER, PH.D.
5110 DALECARLIA DRIVE
BETHESDA, MARYLAND 20816

March 26, 2001

RECEIVED
APR - 9 2001

Dr. C.W. Jameson
National Toxicology Program
Report on Carcinogens
MD EC-14 P.O. Box 12233
Research Triangle Park, NC 27709

Dear Dr. Jameson.

I write in support of the listing of steroidal estrogens in the National Toxicology Program's Report on Carcinogens, Tenth Edition.

Steroidal estrogens are known carcinogens. The International Agency for Research on Cancer (IARC) has reported for some time that a large body of evidence in both animal models and humans demonstrates that estrogens cause cancer.

All of us are exposed to estrogens in numerous forms, from animal feed additives to the xenoestrogens in herbicides, pesticides, and plastics. However, women bear a larger burden of exogenous estrogen exposure throughout the life course. From adolescence when estrogens are prescribed for menstrual irregularities and contraception, to childbearing and the use of estrogens to suppress lactation, and to the use of hormone replacement therapy for menopause and osteoporosis, women in industrialized countries have for many years been exposed to significantly higher levels of exogenous estrogens than men.

In particular, according to the National Center for Health Statistics more than 10.4 million U.S. women used oral contraceptives in 1995. A recent article in the Washington Post reported that 8.6 million menopausal women use combination hormone replacement therapy while an additional 12 million women use unopposed estrogren replacement therapy (Washington Post, March 26, 2001). Many women's health activists and others have argued against the widespread use of both these estrogen products, in part because good alternatives are readily available. Samuel Epstein, M.D. has said, "Worldwide use of birth control pills, in spite of conclusive evidence or carcinogenicity of estrogens in experimental animals, constitutes the largest uncontrolled experiment in human carcinogenesis ever undertaken" (Epstein, 1998, 141).

Of particular concern to all women is the possible link between estrogens and breast cancer. More than 182,000 U.S. women are diagnosed each year with invasive breast cancer and more than 40,000 die annually from the disease (American Cancer Society, 2000). In 1940 an

American woman's lifetime risk of breast cancer was 1 in 20. By 1960, the lifetime risk had risen to 1 in 14. By 1988, the risk was 1 in 10 and within a few short years the risk became 1 woman in 8 (Rinzler, 1993).

The risk of breast cancer due to estrogen use increases with length of use, dose amount, and repeated exposures to estrogen. A meta-analysis of more than 50,000 women with breast cancer, reported in *The Lancet* in 1997, demonstrated that the use of hormone replacement therapy (HRT) for 4 years resulted in an excess of one woman with breast cancer for every 1000 woman users. Use of HRT for 13 years resulted in an excess of one woman with breast cancer for every 100 users (Sherman, 2000).

Breast cancer has become a modern day scourge for women, with no clear understanding of its causes or ways to prevent it. In addition to justified concerns regarding steroidal estrogens is the proliferation of xenoestrogens in the larger environment in which we all live. In other words, the context of women's estrogen exposure has, in recent decades, grown far larger than women's own hormone production or the estrogen-containing medications prescribed to women during their lifetimes. As Sandra Steingraber, Ph.D. has pointed out, "Xenoestrogens not only mimic natural estrogens directly but also can indirectly enhance their effects" (in Kasper and Ferguson, 2000, 288). A recent newsletter of the Cornell University Program on Breast Cancer and Environmental Risk Factors in New York State reports on the "alarming increase" of premature thelarche, or premature sexual development among children in Puerto Rico. The authors pose the question of whether estrogenic environmental contaminants are the cause of this phenomenon.

There is at present no way to determine the effects of the full range of accumulated estrogen exposures in the bodies of individual women. The widespread presence of estrogens, their carcinogenic properties, and the epidemic of breast cancer are much-needed and important areas for further research. Furthermore, the most recent issue of the *Journal of the American Medical Association* reports on a 14-year study supported by the American Cancer Society of more than 211,000 women that demonstrated a 2.2 fold increase in the rate of ovarian cancer for women who had taken estrogens for more than 10 years (*JAMA*, March 21, 2001). While we have known about the association of HRT with endometrial cancer and breast cancer, evidence of the link between HRT and ovarian cancer has not been reported until now.

In the interest of protecting the health of all women, the Second World Conference on Breast Cancer adopted the Precautionary Principle, calling for no substance to be released into the environment until its safety has been established (Second World Conference on Breast Cancer, 1999). Listing steroidal estrogens is a wise step towards safeguarding women's health and perhaps reducing the incidence of breast and other cancers.

Yours truly,

Anne S. Kasper Ph.D

Anne S. Kasper, Ph.D.
Senior Research Scientist

NATIONAL WOMEN'S HEALTH NETWORK

April 16, 2001

Dr. C.W. Jameson
National Toxicology Program
Report on Carcinogens
MD EC-14
P.O. Box 12233
Research Triangle Park, NC 27709

Dear Dr. Jameson:

I am writing on behalf of the National Women's Health Network to commend you and the National Toxicology Program for your decision to include steroidal estrogens in the Tenth Edition of the Report on Carcinogens.

The National Women's Health Network is the only membership-based women's organization that advocates on behalf of the health of all women. Founded in 1975, the Network's mission is to advocate for national policies that protect and promote all women's health and to provide evidence-based, independent information to empower women to make fully informed health decisions. The Network is committed to acting as an independent voice for women's health and thus accepts no money from companies that sell pharmaceuticals, medical devices, dietary supplements, alcohol, tobacco, or health insurance.

While the Network is well aware of the constructive uses of steroid estrogens in medicine and we do not oppose all such uses, we are also very concerned about the cancer risks posed by the drug. Since our founding we have worked to ensure that women will be provided with accurate and complete information about the risks posed by drugs prescribed for them. One of our first policy actions taken when the organization was founded was to advocate for the inclusion of information for patients about the health risks associated with drugs containing estrogen.

More than 25 years later, health risks associated with estrogen are still of significant concern to the organization. Premarin, a steroidal estrogen marketed for hormone replacement therapy at menopause, is the most prescribed drug in the United States. The drug is approved for use in treating hot flashes and osteoporosis, but it also has been found to be associated with an increased risk of breast, endometrial and ovarian cancer. The association of estrogen use with endometrial cancer has been known and acknowledged for many years. Women who use estrogen are twice as likely to develop endometrial cancer than women who have never used hormones. In January 1999, a long-term cohort study of participants in the Breast Cancer Detection Demonstration Project found an increased risk of breast cancer with estrogen-progestin therapy over that associated with estrogen therapy. And in March 2001, the

Founders · Barbara Seaman · Phyllis Chesler, Ph.D. · Belita Cowan · Alice Wolfson · Mary Howell, M.D

The only national public-interest membership organization devoted solely to women and health
514 10th Street, N.W., Ste. 400, Washington, D.C. 20004 • (202) 347-1140 • Fax (202) 347-1168
http://www.womenshealthnetwork.org

American Cancer Society (ACS) reported the results of a study showing that the risk of ovarian cancer also doubled with long-term use of estrogen.

Based on our fundamental commitment to the principal that with accurate and complete information women can make good health decisions for themselves, we believe it is critically important that health care providers and other medical professionals acknowledge the risks associated with steroidal estrogens and share this information with their patients. Including this class of drugs in the Tenth Edition of the Report on Carcinogens is an important step in this direction.

Thank you for the opportunity to comment on the proposed listing. If you have any questions regarding our comments, please do not hesitate to contact me. I can be reached at the offices of the National Women's Health Network:

514 Tenth Street, NW
Fourth Floor
Washington, DC 20004
T: 202.347.1140
F: 202.347.1168
E: aallina@womenshealthnetwork.org

Thank you.

Sincerely,

Amy Allina
Program & Policy Director

Jameson.Bill

From: SSMoench@aol.com
Sent: Friday, May 18, 2001 4:22 PM
To: Jameson.Bill
Subject: Breast cancer

sssDear Dr. Jameson:

I am a physician in Salt Lake City, Utah. My 28 yr. old daughter was diagnosed with breast cancer a year ago and ended up having a double mastectomy last September. Obviously our whole family has been devasted but also shocked because she has absolutely no family history of breast or any other cancer. She was eventually tested for the BCRA gene which was negative. In the course of looking up studies on the National Cancer Institute web site to try and help determine what treatment she needed I came across an overwhelming body of evidence that linked breast cancer in young women with birth control pill use. My daughter had used the pill for 10 yrs. It is the only explanation for her cancer.

I understand that you are receiving public comment about whether the National Toxicology Panel should place estrogen on the list of known carcinogens. In view of what has happened to our family I urge you recommend that estrogen be placed on that list.

It seems that the medical research community spends a great deal of effort, time and money pursuing treatments for cancer and far less on finding the causes. When we do find something that seems to be a cause we have an obligation to warn society even if it is socially or economically unwelcome news. I am sure that the pharmaceutical industry does not want to tarnish the profitability of birth control pills and estrogen replacement therapy. However, the evidence should compel physicians to start warning the public about the dangers of their use. I have watched with particular dismay a recent TV ad campaign encouraging young women to use the pill for such things as regulating their periods and curing acne. Physicians must stand up against the pharmaceutical industry when they endanger the public. This is your chance to do just that and I hope you will.

Sincerely,

Dr. Brian Moench
Salt Lake City, Utah

NAMS
THE NORTH AMERICAN MENOPAUSE SOCIETY

March 1, 2002
By FedEx

RECEIVED
MAR 4 2002

C. W. Jameson, PhD
NTP/NIEHS
79TW Alexander Drive
Building 4401, Room 3118
Research Triangle Park, NC 27709

Dear Dr. Jameson:

We submit this letter as a Task Force convened by the Board of Trustees of The North American Menopause Society (NAMS). NAMS is a nonprofit scientific organization dedicated to promoting women's health during midlife and beyond through the understanding of menopause. Its multidisciplinary membership of 2,000 leaders in the field – including clinical and basic science experts from medicine, nursing, sociology, psychology, nutrition, anthropology, epidemiology, and education – allows NAMS to be among the world's most trusted resources on all aspects of menopause to healthcare providers, researchers, and the public.

We commend the National Toxicology Program (NTP) for its ongoing mission to identify potential and known human carcinogens. However, we are concerned regarding its decision to include natural steroidal estrogens as "known human carcinogens" in the Tenth Report on Carcinogens.

The NTP's Clay B. Frederick, PhD, an invited speaker at the last Annual Meeting of The North American Menopause Society (October 3-5, 2001), encouraged us to submit our comments. At this conference, over 1,400 participants enjoyed the debate – "Estrogen Is/Is Not a Carcinogen" – in which Dr. Frederick presented the NTP's findings. We have been assured by Dr. Frederick and your office that our comments will be considered, although the deadline for comments has passed.

COMMENTS

Including natural steroidal estrogens as "known human carcinogens" is a weighty step for the panel -- one that has great potential for harm to American women. **It should not be taken on the evidence presently available. The definition of a carcinogen that the NTP uses requires a <u>causal</u> relationship between the agent and human cancer. But, only an <u>association</u> with human cancer has been shown. Evidence of a causal effect remains unproven.**

Location
5900 Landerbrook Drive
Suite 195
Mayfield Heights, OH 44124

Mailing Address
Post Office Box 94527
Cleveland, OH 44101-4527

Telephone: 440/442 7550
Fax: 440/442-2660
E-Mail: info@menopause.org
Web Site: http://www.menopause.org

We have similar concern regarding the listing of several hormones in past editions as reasonably anticipated to be a human carcinogen" (eg, 17β-estradiol, progesterone) and "known to be a human carcinogen" (eg, components of conjugated estrogens).

We are concerned about the millions of women who may be confused, harmed, or alarmed by this action of the NTP. We respectfully ask the NTP not to declare steroidal estrogens as "known human carcinogens." In addition, we hope that endogenous human hormones (eg, 17β-estradiol, progesterone) will be reviewed for possible removal from the list of "reasonably anticipated to be a human carcinogen."

Should the NTP add steroidal estrogens to the list of "known human carcinogens," we urge consideration to using some type of grading scale. To place steroidal hormones on the same risk level as sulfites is inappropriate. Even putting diethylstilbestrol on the list does not meet the 1996 Federal guidelines as the relationship between DES and cancer has not been proven to be other than the disruption of the genital development program in such as manner as to open retained fetal genital cells to carcinogens.

To support our position, we offer the *Proposed Guidelines for Carcinogen Risk Assessment*, as published in the *Federal Register* on April 23, 1996 (Federal Register: 17960-18011) (copy attached). These are a revision of EPA's 1986 guidelines, as a better understanding of the actions of carcinogens had been obtained during the prior decade. We would like to call to your attention the following four points from the 1996 document:

Point 1. *"The 1986 cancer guidelines have several limitations in addition to their inadequacy in addressing recent gains in the understanding of carcinogenesis. Although they called for the evaluation of all relevant information, the classification scheme used for identifying potential human hazard relied heavily on tumor findings, and in practice, seldom made full use of all biological information." ... "Hazard assessment emphasizes analysis of all biological information rather than just tumor findings."* Our comments on this point:

This practice of not making full use of all biological information, and not disclosing it objectively, continued with the present report(s). **To date, no studies have unequivocally shown induction of any type of cancer by estrogens.**

A. Estrogen and Endometrial Cancer

Epidemiological studies generally show an association or relative risk, not causal relationships. No cause-effect relationship of estrogen to <u>any</u> cancer can be drawn from available epidemiological studies, and no attempts should be made to draw such conclusions. Therefore, all epidemiological studies quoted by the Committee are not interpretable by the NTP's own definition. To the contrary, steroidal estrogens and many other tested estrogen receptor ligands have never been shown by direct testing to be carcinogens. This includes both animal and human testing. Ergo, the risk of estrogen-induced cancer should be small – and it is.

The association between estrogen replacement therapy (ERT) and "endometrial cancer" is dubious. At the time of the initial reports of a relationship of ERT to endometrial cancer, it was stated repeatedly that the excess number of diagnosed cases were of low (nuclear) grade. The clear clinical difference between low nuclear grade endometrial cancer (LGED) and high nuclear grade endometrial cancer (HGEC) was not known. Both were thought to be part of the continuum toward a single entity; LGEC and HGEC were referred to as "low grade" and "high grade" endometrial adenocarcinoma, respectively. This is important because the diagnosis of extreme atypical hyperplasia vs. LGEC may be very subjective, and the biological outcomes are generally innocent.

In fact, LGEC and HGEC have different characteristics and outcomes, namely, LGEC almost always is estrogen-receptor positive (ER+), is hormonally responsive, rarely metastasizes, and is almost always cured by progestogen treatment or removal of the tumor in the uterus. In contrast, HGEC generally lacks estrogen receptors and is, therefore, insensitive to hormones, metastasizes early, and is often fatal if not diagnosed before metastases occur.

Since previously it was thought that one lesion blended into the other (LGE → HGEC), the main effort was placed on early diagnosis rather than separating the two entities. In fact, definitive early diagnosis of LGEC remains difficult since there is a continuum of benign hyperplasia, cytological atypia, and malignant change to be interpreted.

Since the addition of anti-estrogenic progestogens to ERT in women with intact uteri (the combination called hormone replacement therapy or HRT) obviates the occurrence of LGEC, progestogen use has become the clinical standard. The inflated number of diagnosed "endometrial cancers" has fallen and become of relatively small interest to gynecologists. But, the rate of HGEC has not diminished and its sporadic and uncommon occurrence have put HGEC "below the radar" of the methods being used to evaluate the question of HRT's effect on endometrial cancer. Nonetheless, a clue to this issue is found in the evidence that a woman using HRT at the time of diagnosis of "endometrial cancer" has no demonstrable different in lifespan as compared to non-ERT users.

Unfortunately, there have been few efforts to sort these matters out in light of the current understanding of endometrial cancer and there is no resolution to whether the association of estrogen with endometrial cancer (HGEC, to be precise) is causal or casual. Rather, ignorance has prevailed and few understand that only an association has been proven, **and that association is with LGEC and not HGEC.**

A few clinical trials of low-to-modest-dose ERT in women with uteri have begun to appear that show no increase in endometrial cancer. Hopefully, they will help spur the reconsideration of the relationship of ERT to endometrial cancer that is so long overdue.

As responsible clinicians, we are concerned about the potential association between unopposed estrogen and endometrial cancer that was suggested in past epidemiological studies. These concerns led to advising cautious use of estrogen therapy in postmenopausal women with an intact uterus. We continue doing so until such time when well-controlled, prospective studies have established whether there is a link between endometrial cancer and contemporary estrogen therapy. However, the time-honored approach of adding anti-estrogenic progestogens to ERT is not based on biological evidence directly linking contemporary estrogen and endometrial cancer, since these data are lacking.

B. Estrogen and Breast Cancer

In order to understand the issues as they pertain to breast cancer, it is necessary to distinguish between the evidence associating locally-formed estrogen with breast cancer and the lack of evidence associating ERT/HRT with the incidence of breast cancer.

None of the epidemiological studies linking estrogen and/or progestogen treatment (ie, ERT/HRT) with breast cancer that were quoted by the Committee are biologically applicable to the NTP's definition of a carcinogen. There is more likelihood that the relationship of estrogen to breast cancer is in need of objective re-evaluation. In short, the contemporary evidence indicates that estrogen, but not ERT/HRT, is associated with adenocarcinoma for the breast. The nature of that association is not known. Evidence indicates that the local production of estrogen in the breast is the major determinant in that relationship. This casts doubt on the idea that the doses of hormone in contemporary ERT could be a material factor, if at all involved in the etiology of breast cancer.

The picture is further complicated by many issues, namely (1) the precise nature of the cancer(s) at issue is not known, (2) the length of residence of small numbers of malignant cells in the breasts and their trajectory through *in situ* to metastatic disease is not known, (3) the impact of rapid improvement of early diagnostic methods that has occurred during the same period, (4) the role of surviving past other diseases that might have claimed study subjects earlier, and (5) hormone effects on other systems in aging individuals.

At present, the available evidence shows: (1) improved prognosis if one is using ERT when the breast cancer is diagnosed, (2) that estrogens (including DES) are effective treatments for breast cancer, and (3) no increase is seen in recurrences of breast cancer in tumor-free women who receive ERT for symptoms. All are contradictory to the idea that ERT/HRT cause breast cancer and fit with the idea of a relationship including exposure of sensitive cells in the breast to factors leading to breast cancer, including locally formed estrogen.

How the locally-formed estrogen is related: The Committee apparently did not seriously consider the possibility that the issue of direct versus indirect actions of estrogen may be the result of activation of signaling cascades distal to the effect of estrogen, each of which can promote tumor progression by itself. Notable among them are growth factors and oncogenes, all of which relate to cancer biology. At present, relatively little is known about cancer induction and initiation in general, and even less about the effects of estrogen. In the recent Committee report, recommendations were based on non-epidemiological studies, using animal models or tissue cultures. Conditions preclude drawing conclusions of direct cause-effect of estrogen. For instance, in experiments done in the presence of serum or oncogenes, the "cancer-promoting effect of estrogen" can be due to estrogen-induced increased sensitivity of the cell to the oncogene or simply the increased proliferation of cells that opens the genome to malignant transformation. Thus, an erroneous conclusion can be drawn that estrogen is a carcinogen, while in reality, oncogenes or other agents are the tumor initiators.

Point 2. *"Hazard characterization is added to integrate the data analysis of all relevant studies into a weight of evidence conclusion of hazard, to develop a working conclusion regarding the agent's mode of action in leading to tumor development, and to describe the conditions under which the hazard may be expressed (eg, route, pattern, duration, and magnitude of exposure)."* Our comments on this point:

Scientifically, it is hazardous to integrate data from different experiments into one body of a "working conclusion." In fact, a single well-designed study may have a greater biological significance than many weak studies. Combining data from a number of studies into meta-analyses has questionable scientific merit, and is dismissed *a priori* by knowledgeable scholars in biology and medicine.

However, this issue is even more complicated because in the path of revealing the "truth," one may often encounter conflicting results obtained from well-designed studies. For instance, two well-designed and well-conducted studies tested the same hypothesis, whether tamoxifen can prevent breast cancer, namely, the NSABP P-1 (Dunn BK, Ford LG. Breast cancer prevention: results of the National Surgical Adjuvant Breast and Bowel Project (NSABP) breast cancer prevention trial (NSABP P-1:BCPT). *Eur J Cancer* 2000;36:S49-50) and the Royal Marsden Hospital trial (Powles TJ, et al. The Royal Marsden Hospital pilot tamoxifen chemoprevention trial. *Breast Cancer Res Treat* 1994;31:73-82). Interestingly, they came to entirely different conclusions.

Therefore, while no one single study may have monopoly over the "truth" of whether estrogen is a carcinogen, truth can be ascertained only when sufficient numbers of appropriate studies are conducted. As was stated above, at present no appropriate studies have been conducted to unequivocally determine the cause-effect of estrogen and cancer in humans.

Point 3. *The sections about "Dose response assessment is a two-step process" and "Three default approaches: Linear, nonlinear, or both."* Our comments on this point:

We understand from these paragraphs that the Committee's key argument is that of deriving secondary data (dose-response results) and turning it into prime evidence. This is similar to meta-analysis; by using secondary data from initially faulted or irrelevant studies, one cannot derive "stronger" conclusions.

Point 4. *"Descriptions of major default assumptions and criteria for departing from them are described." ... "Risk characterization is more fully developed by providing direction on how the overall conclusions and confidence of risk is presented for the risk manager. The Proposed Guidelines call for assumptions and uncertainties to be clearly explained."* Our comments on this point:

We assume that appropriate, objective, scientifically sound, self-criticism of the Committee's final statements has occurred. In support of such a serious and precedent-setting decision, these discussions should be presented for evaluation by the lay and medical public.

In addition, we have not seen the alternative hypotheses proposed by the Committee as to how estrogen could increase the risk of cancer. For instance, estrogen may prolong life and, thereby, the risk of cancer in women. The risk of breast cancer increases with age, and if a woman lives long enough, she increases her risk of developing breast cancer. Thus, it is possible that the increased incidence of breast cancer reported in some epidemiological studies of postmenopausal women treated with estrogen depends on longevity rather than on estrogen.

Another example: estrogen is a mitogen. Dividing cells, especially in older persons (both men and women), are more susceptible to *de-novo* chromosomal malfunctions that may lead to neoplasia. Therefore, it is possible that the increased incidence reported in some epidemiological studies of endometrial and breast cancer in postmenopausal women treated with estrogen depends on enhanced cell division, rather than on estrogen.

In Conclusion

In short, the evidence is that estrogen's relationship to the two most often cited cancers is that of an association, and not a causative effect. There is no evidence to indicate, much less confirm, that estrogen is a direct carcinogen. The argument of those in favor of using the association of a naturally-secreted hormone such as estrogen to identify those substances as carcinogens appears to be the beginning of a slippery slope which ultimately will lead to the identification of all mitogens as carcinogens.

While scientists who have great knowledge of the subject may comfortably disagree on whether estrogen is a carcinogen, imagine the burden that such a label places on the average woman who has natural exposure to a compound labeled as a carcinogen, or is considering ERT. Perhaps one day evidence will resolve this issue. Until then, surely we do a disservice to both our patients and our profession (clinicians and scientists) when we allow imprecision and selective observations to cloud the central evidence in these issues.

While ignorance may be a defense against our failure to fully resolve the role of estrogen in endometrial cancer and the effects that those reports had on women in the 1970s, the issues about which we are ignorant at this time are apparent. We must resist premature use of terms that likely will do greater harm than good. *"Primum non nocere"* is quite an apt motto in this issue.

The health consequences of the NTP's actions on these hormones are significant. Should you wish to continue this discussion, and/or should you wish a list of references for this material, please contact NAMS at 440/442-7550. Should you desire, we would also be pleased to provide an electronic file of this letter for posting on the NTB Web site.

Sincerely,

Carcinogen Task Force
The North American Menopause Society

George I. Gorodeski, MD, PhD
Associate Professor of Reproductive Biology, and
Physiology and Biophysics
Case Western Research University School of Medicine
University Hospitals of Cleveland
Cleveland, OH

Frederick Naftolin, MD, DPhil
Professor, Department of Obstetrics and Gynecology
Yale University School of Medicine
New Haven, CT

Wulf H. Utian, MD, PhD
Arthur H. Bill Professor Emeritus of
Reproductive Biology, and Obstetrics and Gynecology
Case Western Reserve University School of Medicine
Consultant in Women's Health
Cleveland Clinic
Cleveland, OH

From: Barbara
Sent: Thursday, October 18, 2001 07:56 AM
To: jameson@niehs.nih.gov
Subject: NAMS Drug Company Sponsors

RECEIVE
OCT 18 2001

October 18, 2001

To: Dr. C.W. Jameson
National Toxicology Program
Report on Carcinogens
P.O. Box 12233
79 Alexander Drive
Bldg.4401, Room 3127, MD-EC-14
Research Triangle Park, NC 27709

Dear Dr. Jameson,

I hope it is not to late to ask that this note be added to the comments supporting the National Toxicology Program's decision to include steroidal estrogens in the Tenth Edition of the Report on Carcinogens. I write in response to an an Oct 8, 2001 Reuters Health News article entitled "Listing of Estrogen as 'Known Carcinogen' Hotly Debated." The article, which appears on Medscape, states that at the 12th annual meeting of the North American Menopause Society (NAMS), Dr. Clay B. Frederick, a member of the National Toxicology Program presented the case for considering estrogen as a carcinogen, while Dr. James V. Fiorica of the H. Lee Moffitt Cancer Center in Tampa spoke for the opposition. The Reuters article begins with the statement, "Members of the North American Menopause Society are protesting the move to add estrogen to the list of human carcinogens compiled by the National Institute of Environmental Health Sciences." It concludes with the statement, "Dr. Wolf Utian, executive director of NAMS, said his group is considering submitting a formal response to the RoC."

NAMS is a well- respected organization, and Dr. Fiorica of the H. Lee Moffitt Cancer Center in Tampa is a well-respected physician. However, both appear to have financial ties with hormone manufacturers, and I ask that this potential conflict-of-interest be presented alongside any commentary the NAMS may submit. According to its own website, NAMS, a nonprofit organization, has eighteen current corporate "Partners in Menopause." Here is the list:

"NAMS Partners in Menopause

NAMS wishes to acknowledge the following 18 companies for their participation in the Partners in Menopause Education program for 2001. These companies are loyal supporters that actively participate in evaluating ways in which the mission of the Society can be better achieved.

Allergan
Berlex Laboratories
Eli Lilly and Company
GlaxoSmithKline Consumer Healthcare
LDS Consumer Products
Merck & Co.
Monarch Pharmaceuticals, Inc. Women's Health
Novogen Inc.
Novogyne Pharmaceuticals
Organon, Inc.
Ortho-McNeil Pharmaceutical, Inc.
Pfizer
Pharmacia Corporation
Procter & Gamble Pharmaceuticals
Protein Technologies International
SmithKline Beecham Consumer Healthcare
Solvay Pharmaceuticals, Inc.
Warner-Chilcott
Wyeth-Ayerst Pharmaceuticals

Contents © 2001 The North American Menopause Society. All rights reserved."

At the same New Orleans meeting where NAMS disputed the carcinogenicity of estrogen, it presented three research grants of $20,000 each conjointly with pharmaceutical companies, one with Solvay and two with Wyeth-Ayeerst.

In addition six awards of merit were awarded conjointly with Pfizer, Organon, Protein Technologies, Eli Lilly (2) and Ortho-McNeil. In addition, the NAMS/Wyeth-Ayerst Nurse Practitioner Reporter Program recognized 10 outstanding nurse practitioners. As for Dr. Fiorica, he contributed to a recently-expired (August 31) Continuing Medical Education (CME) Medscape Women's Health Treatment Update called "Straight Talk on HRT: Benefits and Limitations." This continuing education tool for medical professionals is "Supported by an unrestricted educational grant from Wyeth-Ayerst Laboratories."

On a second matter, I wish to note that any continuing debate on the role of estrogen in cancer usually centers on the breast. There can be no debate whatsoever as to the role of estrogens in promoting cancer of the endometrium. This was assumed to be the case since 1947, and confirmed to the full satisfaction of FDA in 1975. Back in the December, 1947 issue of The American Journal of Obstetrics and Gynecology, Dr. Saul Gusberg (later to be president of the American Cancer Society) published a report of 29 patients whose endometria were profoundly disturbed by estrogen therapy prescribed in menopause,- 20 with hyperplasia, nine with cancer. In December, 1975, following the publication of five high-quality studies from independent investigator-groups (see Zeil and Finkle, Kaiser-Permanente, Los Angeles; Donald Smith et al, University of Washington, Seattle; Thomas Mack et al, University of Southern California; Donald Austin, California Tumor Registry; Stadel and Weiss, National Institutes of Health,) the FDA concluded that- "The probability that endometrial cancer will occur in a postmenopausal woman with an intact uterus who does not take estrogen is 1 in 1,000 a year. The risk among estrogen users is 4 to 8 in 1,000 a year, or higher, depending on length of use." In 1991 the author of this letter, among several other women's health advocates, petitioned Dr. Bernadine Healy to redesign the NIH Women's Health Initiative study so that it would not expose women with intact uteri to unopposed estrogens. Dr. Healy responded she'd been advised that such cancers could be averted with careful monitoring. Unfortunately, she was wrong. As SCIENCE MAGAZINE reported in Vol 269, August 11, 1995,-three years after Dr. Healy dismissed our concerns,- the study arm that we objected to was "quietly dropped." (See "Women's Health Research Blosssoms" by Charles Mann, p.766–770.)

I have been covering hormone products as a major part of my science-writer beat since 1960. I have written three books and hundreds of articles on hormones and related topics. I interviewed most of the key scientists who developed estrogens or estrogen applications all the way back to Sir Charles Dodds, and Dr. John Rock. Based on all of the evidence and research I have been following the past 40 years, I believe the decision to include Estrogens as a known carcinogen is not only called for but long over due.

Sincerely,

Barbara Seaman
(Journalist and Author)

M.E. Comments:

The comments and letters by some of the citizens are chilling. Only the drug sponsored doctors were willing to ignore the Committee's recommendation that steriodal estrogens be placed on the "10th RoC" as "known human carcinogens". I do not believe that I am an alarmist. However, to use cancer producing agents to avoid menopausal symptoms (hot flashes, night sweats, vaginal dryness, etc.) or for birth control, makes absolutely no sense. At least they have given up their unscientific statements that synthetic HRT lowers risk of breast cancer, ovarian cancer, cardiovascular disease, stroke, gallbladder disease, and atherosclerosis.

CHAPTER IV

WOMEN'S HEALTH INITIATIVE WHI
NATIONAL INSTITUTE OF HEALTH NIH
NATIONAL HEART, LUNG, AND BLOOD INSTITUTE NHLBI

On July 9, 2002 the headlines in many major U.S. newspapers read "The Women's Health Initiative Study Warns - Stop Taking Prempro™" The warning applies to Prempro™, as well as to other high dose combinations of synthetic estrogens and progestins currently being prescribed to over 8,000,000 women. The Women's Health Initiative (WHI) conducted a large federally funded study on synthetic hormone replacement therapy in post menopausal women. This study was abruptly halted because there was an increase in the risk of invasive breast cancer which could only be attributed to the drugs being used in the study. The following are excerpts from the study which appeared in the journal of the American Medical Association.

ଓଃଓଃ

In the *Journal of American Medical Association*; Vol. 288 No. 3, July 17, 2002: 321-333; "Risks and Benefits of Estrogen Plus Progestin in Healthy Postmenopausal Women" Principal Results From the Women's Health Initiative Randomized Controlled Trial Writing Group for the Women's Health Initiative Investigators reports that...

> On May 31, 2002, after a mean of 5.2 years of follow-up, the data and safety monitoring board recommended stopping the trial of estrogen plus progestin vs placebo because the test statistic for invasive breast cancer exceeded the stopping boundary for this adverse effect and the global index statistic supported risks exceeding benefits.

and concluded that the . . .

> Overall health risks exceeded benefits from use of combined estrogen plus progestin for an average 5.2-year follow-up among healthy postmenopausal US women.

in further commenting they said . . .

> The WHI provides evidence from a large randomized trial that addresses the important issue of whether most women with an intact uterus in the decades of life following menopause should consider hormone therapy to prevent chronic disease. The WHI enrolled a cohort of mostly healthy, ethnically diverse women, spanning a large age range (50-79 years at baseline). It is noteworthy that the increased risks for cardiovascular disease and invasive breast cancer were present across racial/ethnic and age strata and were not influenced by the antecedent risk status or prior disease. Hence, the results are likely to be generally

> applicable to healthy women in this age range. At the time the trial was stopped, the increases in numbers of invasive breast cancers, CHD, stroke, and PE made approximately equal contributions to harm in the estrogen plus progestin group compared with placebo, which were not counterbalanced by the smaller reductions in numbers of hip fractures and colorectal cancers.

With regard to overall risks and benefits they said...

> ...At the end of the trial, the global index indicated that there were more harmful than beneficial outcomes in the estrogen plus progestin group vs the placebo group.

Their implications were that . . .

> The WHI trial results provide the first definitive data on which to base treatment recommendations for healthy postmenopausal women with an intact uterus. This trial did not address the short-term risks and benefits of hormones given for the treatment of menopausal symptoms. On the basis of HERS and other secondary prevention trials, the American Heart Association recommended against initiating postmenopausal hormones for the secondary prevention of cardiovascular disease. The American Heart Association made no firm recommendation for primary prevention

while awaiting the results from randomized clinical trials such as WHI, and stated that continuation of the treatment should be considered on the basis of established noncoronary benefits and risks, possible coronary benefits and risks, and patient preference.

Results from WHI indicate that the combined postmenopausal hormones CEE, 0.625 mg/d, plus MPA, 2.5 mg/d, should not be initiated or continued for the primary prevention of CHD. In addition, the substantial risks for cardiovascular disease and breast cancer must be weighed against the benefit for fracture in selecting from the available agents to prevent osteoporosis.

In an accompanying Editorial titled "Failure of Estrogen Plus Progestin Therapy for Prevention" Suzanne W. Fletcher, MD, MSc; Graham A. Colditz, MD, DrPH write that. . .

Approximately 38% of postmenopausal women in the United States use hormone replacement therapy. In 2000, 46 million prescriptions were written for Premarin® (conjugated estrogens), making it the second most frequently prescribed medication in the United States and accounting for more than $1 billion in sales, and 22.3 million prescriptions were written for Prempro™ (conjugated estrogens plus medroxyprogesterone acetate). . .

. . . Now, the surprising results of the Women's Health Initiative (WHI) are reported in this issue of THE JOURNAL. The WHI is the first randomized primary prevention trial of postmenopausal hormones, and the part of the study that compared estrogen/progestin with placebo was terminated early.

. . .Overall, the results of the WHI study are consistent with the growing body of literature on the effects of combination estrogen/progestin. The increasing risk of breast cancer with duration of use and the reductions in risk of colon cancer and fractures are in the expected direction and magnitude. Risk for stroke and venous thromboembolism continued throughout the 5 years of therapy, whereas the elevated risk of coronary heart disease was largely limited to the first year of therapy. . .

. . .the whole purpose of healthy women taking long-term estrogen/progestin therapy is to preserve health and prevent disease. The results of this study provide strong evidence that the opposite is happening for important aspects of women's health, even if the absolute risk is low. Given these results, we recommend that clinicians stop prescribing this combination for long-term use. Primum non nocere applies especially to preventive health care. The results are for a single dosing regimen (1 daily tablet containing 0.625 mg of conjugated equine estrogen plus 2.5 mg of medroxyprogesterone acetate) and other regimens may have different results, but the 3 studies reported to date in the United States with other regimens have all found an increased risk of breast cancer.

. . . **The WHI provides an important health answer for generations of healthy postmenopausal women to come do not use estrogen/progestin to prevent chronic disease.**

Excerpts from the Women's Health Initiative from their Website

http://www.nhlbi.nih.gov/whi/

NIH News Release of NHLBI Stops Trial of Estrogen Plus Progestin Due to Increased Breast Cancer Risk, Lack of Overall Benefit

Estrogen Plus Progestin Study Stopped Due to Increased Breast Cancer Risk, Lack of Overall Benefit - Questions and Answers

News from the NCI - Questions and Answers: Use of Hormones After Menopause http://www.nhlbi.nih.gov/new/press/02-07-09.htm

NATIONAL INSTITUTES OF HEALTH

National Heart, Lung, and Blood Institute

NIH NEWS RELEASE

EMBARGOED FOR RELEASE
Tuesday, July 9, 2002
9:30 a.m. Eastern Time

Contact:
NHLBI Communications Office:
(301) 496-4236
NCI Press Office: (301) 496-6641

NHLBI STOPS TRIAL OF ESTROGEN PLUS PROGESTIN DUE TO INCREASED BREAST CANCER RISK, LACK OF OVERALL BENEFIT

The National Heart, Lung, and Blood Institute (NHLBI) of the National Institutes of Health (NIH) has stopped early a major clinical trial of the risks and benefits of combined estrogen and progestin in healthy menopausal women due to an increased risk of invasive breast cancer. The large multi-center trial, a component of the Women's Health Initiative (WHI), also found increases in coronary heart disease, stroke, and pulmonary embolism in study participants on estrogen plus progestin compared to women taking placebo pills. There were noteworthy benefits of estrogen plus progestin, including fewer cases of hip fractures and colon cancer, but on balance the harm was greater than the benefit. The study, which was scheduled to run until 2005, was stopped after an average follow-up of 5.2 years.

Participants in this component of WHI, like most women with a uterus who take hormone therapy, were given progestin in combination with estrogen. This practice is known to prevent endometrial cancer. A separate WHI study of estrogen alone in women who had a hysterectomy before joining the WHI hormone program continues unchanged because, at this point, the balance of risks and benefits of estrogen alone is still uncertain.

The report from the WHI investigators on the estrogen plus progestin study findings will be published in the July 17 issue of *The Journal of the American Medical Association (JAMA)*; because of the importance of the information, the study is being released early on Tuesday, July 9, as an expedited article on the *JAMA* Web site. (Full text version available to all at jama.com.)

"We have long sought the answer to the question: Does postmenopausal hormone therapy prevent heart disease and, if it does, what are the risks? The bottom-line answer from WHI is that this combined form of hormone therapy is unlikely to benefit the heart. The cardiovascular and cancer risks of estrogen plus progestin outweigh any benefits--and a 26 percent increase in breast cancer risk is too high a price to pay, even if there were a heart benefit. Similarly, the risks outweigh the benefits of fewer hip fractures," said NHLBI Director Claude Lenfant, M.D.

"Menopausal women who might have been candidates for estrogen plus progestin should now focus on well-proven treatments to reduce the risk of cardiovascular disease, including measures to prevent and control high blood pressure, high blood cholesterol, and obesity. This effort could not be more important: heart disease remains the number one killer of American women," added Lenfant.

The estrogen plus progestin trial of the WHI involved 16,608 women ages 50 to 79 years with an intact uterus. An important objective of the trial was to examine the effect of estrogen plus progestin on the prevention of heart disease and hip fractures, and any associated change in risk for breast and colon cancer. The study did not address the short-term risks and benefits of hormones for the treatment of menopausal symptoms.

About 6 million women in the U.S. are taking estrogen plus progestin for a variety of reasons, including symptom relief, because their doctors advised it, or for long-term health.

"Women with a uterus who are currently taking estrogen plus progestin should have a serious talk with their doctor to see if they should continue it. If they are taking this hormone combination for short-term relief of symptoms, it may be reasonable to continue since the benefits are likely to outweigh the risks. Longer term use or use for disease prevention must be re-evaluated given the multiple adverse effects noted in WHI," said Jacques Rossouw, M.D., acting director of the WHI.

According to Rossouw, the adverse effects of estrogen plus progestin applied to all women, irrespective of age, ethnicity, or prior disease status.

"When the estrogen-only trial is completed, a comparison of the results of these two trials may provide a better idea of the roles of estrogen, compared to estrogen plus progestin, in health and disease," said Marcia Stefanick, Ph.D., chair of the WHI Steering

Committee and Associate Professor of Medicine, Stanford University, Palo Alto, California.

Women enrolled in the estrogen plus progestin study were randomly assigned to a daily dose of estrogen plus progestin (0.625 mg of conjugated equine estrogens plus 2.5 mg of medroxyprogesterone acetate) or to a placebo. Participants were enrolled in the study between 1993 and 1998 at over 40 clinical sites across the country.

In 2000 and again in 2001, WHI investigators complied with a recommendation from the study's Data and Safety Monitoring Board (DSMB) to inform participants of a small increase in heart attacks, strokes, and blood clots in women taking hormones. The DSMB, an independent advisory committee charged with reviewing results and ensuring participant safety, found that the actual number of women having any one of these events was small and it did not cross the statistical boundary established to ensure participant safety. Therefore, the group recommended continuing the trial due to the still uncertain balance of risks and benefits.

Then, at the DSMB's regularly scheduled meeting on May 31, 2002, the data review revealed for the first time that the number of cases of invasive breast cancer in the estrogen plus progestin group had crossed the boundary established as a signal of increased risk.

"In designing the trial and following the results, the safety of the patients was of the utmost importance," said Garnet Anderson, Ph.D., a biostatistician who led the analysis at the Fred Hutchinson Cancer Research Center, Seattle, Washington. "Because breast cancer is so serious an event, we set the bar lower to monitor for it. We pre-specified that the change in cancer rates did not have to be that large to warrant stopping the trial. And the trial was stopped at the first clear indication of increased risk," she added. She also noted that, at that point, there was no indication of increased risk for breast cancer in the estrogen-only group.

The DSMB's May 31 recommendation to stop the trial was based on the finding of increased breast cancer risk, supported by the evidence of overall health risks exceeding any benefits. Following the NHLBI's decision to stop the study, the Institute and the investigators have worked intensively to develop information materials for participants. On July 8, participants started receiving letters informing them about the results and telling them that they should stop study medications. Participants will be contacted by their clinical centers for further counseling and will continue to have clinic visits so that their health outcomes can be followed.

All WHI participants, including those in the other study components, are also receiving a newsletter with a summary of the findings and an explanation of risks and benefits.

Dr. Rossouw stressed the importance of understanding how the risk to an individual woman can be low, but the risk to the population at large can be great.

"The WHI results tell us that during 1 year, among 10,000 postmenopausal women with a uterus who are taking estrogen plus progestin, 8 more will have invasive breast cancer, 7 more will have a heart attack, 8 more will have a stroke, and 18 more will have blood clots, including 8 with blood clots in the lungs, than will a similar group of 10,000 women not taking these hormones. This is a relatively small annual increase in risk for an individual woman. Individual women who have participated in the trial and women in the population who have been on estrogen and progestin should not be unduly alarmed. However, even small individual risks over time, and on a population-wide basis, add up to tens of thousands of these serious adverse health events," explained Rossouw.

The National Cancer Institute (NCI) re-emphasized the recommendation that all women in their forties and older get screened for breast cancer with mammography every 1 to 2 years.

"Women in the WHI, women taking hormones for any reason, and any woman over 40 should remain committed to their regular program of breast cancer screening to allow the earliest possible detection of breast cancer," said Leslie Ford, M.D., associate director for clinical research in NCI's Division of Cancer Prevention.

"The reduction in colorectal cancer risk in the WHI is intriguing, but the balance of harm versus benefit does not justify any woman beginning or continuing to take estrogen plus progestin for this purpose. NCI has a number of clinical trials under way investigating new methods to detect and prevent both colorectal cancer and breast cancer that will provide critical information to help women make important health decisions," added Ford.

Specific study findings for the estrogen plus progestin group compared to placebo include:

- A 41 percent increase in strokes
- A 29 percent increase in heart attacks

- A doubling of rates of venous thromboembolism (blood clots)
- A 22 percent increase in total cardiovascular disease
- A 26 percent increase in breast cancer
- A 37 percent reduction in cases of colorectal cancer
- A one-third reduction in hip fracture rates
- A 24 percent reduction in total fractures
- No difference in total mortality (of all causes)

The WHI involves over 161,000 women who are participating in a set of clinical trials or an observational study. The clinical trials are designed to test promising but unproven preventive measures for heart disease, breast and colorectal cancer, and osteoporosis. In addition to the trials of estrogen alone and estrogen plus progestin, other trials are studying a low-fat eating pattern and calcium/Vitamin D supplementation. WHI is sponsored by NHLBI in collaboration with four other components of the NIH-- the National Cancer Institute, the National Institute of Arthritis and Musculoskeletal and Skin Diseases, the National Institute on Aging, and the Office of Research on Women's Health. Note: Wyeth-Ayerst Research provided the medication (active hormones and placebo) for the estrogen plus progestin study.

NATIONAL HEART, LUNG, AND BLOOD INSTITUTE NATIONAL INSTITUTES OF HEALTH

THE WOMEN'S HEALTH INITIATIVE

http://www.nhlbi.nih.gov/whi/index.html

Estrogen Plus Progestin Study Stopped Due to Increased Breast Cancer Risk, Lack of Overall Benefit

Questions and Answers

- What is the purpose of the WHI study on combination hormone therapy?
- Why were the women in the WHI estrogen plus progestin study told to stop study pills at this time?
- What were the main findings in the WHI study on estrogen plus progestin?
- What are the increased risks for women taking estrogen plus progestin?
- What are the reduced risks for women taking estrogen plus progestin?
- What are the conclusions from these findings?
- What were the actual hormones that women in the estrogen plus progestin study were taking?
- When did the increased risk of breast cancer become apparent for women taking estrogen plus progestin compared to women taking placebo pills?
- Is there an increased risk of breast cancer in women taking estrogen alone?

- Is there an increased risk for ovarian cancer with long-term use of estrogen alone?
- How does this new information affect women in the WHI study of estrogen alone?
- Do you have recommendations about other hormone alternatives (lower-dose estrogens, micronized progesterone, natural hormones)?
- I am taking prescription hormones, what should I do?
- Does this new information apply to Selective Estrogen Receptor Modulators (SERMS) or phyto-estrogens?
- How does all of this new information affect my decision to use HRT for relief from hot flashes, sleep problems and mood swings?

Q. What is the purpose of the WHI study on combination hormone therapy?

A. The long-term studies in the WHI were initiated because over the years a number of research studies presented a complicated picture of the risks and benefits of hormone therapy, and its continued use for prevention of cardiovascular diseases was controversial. This situation led the NIH to conduct a large clinical trial of the risks and benefits of hormone therapy. The WHI set out to examine the long-term effect of estrogen plus progestin on the prevention of heart disease and hip fractures, while monitoring for possible increases in risk for breast and colon cancer. The estrogen plus progestin regimen was given to women who have a uterus since progestin is known to protect against endometrial cancer, a known effect of unopposed estrogen. A separate study of estrogen alone in women who had a hysterectomy was also begun.

Q. Why were the women in the WHI estrogen plus progestin study told to stop study pills at this time?

A. In its most recent review of the study data, the WHI Data and Safety Monitoring Board saw an increased risk of breast cancer in women taking estrogen plus progestin. The Board also saw that the previously identified risks for heart attacks, strokes and blood clots to the lungs and legs had persisted. Therefore, in the judgment of the Board, the overall risks outweighed the benefits of taking estrogen plus progestin.

Q. What were the main findings in the WHI study on estrogen plus progestin?

A. The main findings show that compared to women taking placebo pills:

- The number of women who developed breast cancer was *higher* in women taking estrogen plus progestin.

- The numbers of women who developed heart attacks, strokes, or blood clots in the lungs and legs were *higher* in women taking estrogen plus progestin.
- The numbers of women who had hip and other fractures or colorectal cancer were *lower* in women taking estrogen plus progestin.
- There were no differences in the number of women who had endometrial cancer (cancer of the lining of the uterus) or in the number of deaths.

Q. What are the increased risks for women taking estrogen plus progestin?

A. For every 10,000 women taking estrogen plus progestin pills:

- 38 developed breast cancer each year compared to 30 breast cancers for every 10,000 women taking placebo pills each year.
- 37 had a heart attack compared to 30 out of every 10,000 women taking placebo pills.
- 29 had a stroke each year, compared to 21 out of every 10,000 women taking placebo pills.
- 34 had blood clots in the lungs or legs, compared to 16 women out of every 10,000 women taking placebo pills.

Q. What are the reduced risks for women taking estrogen plus progestin?

A. For every 10,000 women taking estrogen plus progestin pills:

- 10 had a hip fracture each year, compared to 15 out of every 10,000 women taking placebo pills each year.
- 10 developed colon cancer each year, compared to 16 out of every 10,000 women taking placebo pills.

Q. What are the conclusions from these findings?

A. The main conclusions are:

- The estrogen plus progestin combination studied in WHI does not prevent heart disease.
- For women taking this estrogen plus progestin combination, the risks (increased breast cancer, heart attacks, strokes, and blood clots in the lungs and legs) outweigh the benefits (fewer hip fractures and colon cancers).

Q. What were the actual hormones that women in the estrogen plus progestin study were taking?

A. Women who were randomized to receive active hormones were taking conjugated equine estrogens 0.625 mg each day and medroxyprogesterone acetate 2.5 mg each day.

This is the most commonly prescribed postmenopausal hormone therapy in the United States for women who have a uterus (used each day by more than six million women).

Q. When did the increased risk of breast cancer become apparent for women taking estrogen plus progestin compared to women taking placebo pills?

A. There was no difference in the development of breast cancer during the first 4 years between women taking estrogen plus progestin and those taking placebo pills. After that time, the numbers began to increase. After an average of 5.2 years, there was an increased risk of breast cancer in women taking estrogen plus progestin compared to those taking placebo pills.

Q. Is there an increased risk of breast cancer in women taking estrogen alone?

A. There is no evidence of an increased risk for breast cancer in women taking active estrogen alone, compared to those taking placebo pills, even after an average of 5.2 years. We do not know whether the long-term effects will differ. The Data Safety and Monitoring Board will continue to review participants' health data every 6 months.

Q. Is there an increased risk for ovarian cancer with long-term use of estrogen alone?

A. An observational study of women who took estrogen alone found that women who used estrogen alone for 10-19 years were twice as likely to develop ovarian cancer as those who did not use postmenopausal hormones. (Absolute number was about 7 cases per 10,000 women years compared to 4.4 per 10,000 women years if estrogens were never used.) If women used estrogen for twenty years or longer, the number increased to 14 per 10,000 person years.

Q. How does this new information affect women in the WHI study of estrogen alone?

A. The Data and Safety Monitoring Board of the WHI will bc reviewing the information about the risks for ovarian cancer and provide their input to the NIH. The NIH will also send letters to the study investigators updating them with information which they can discuss with study participants.

Q. Do you have recommendations about other hormone alternatives (lower-dose estrogens, micronized progesterone, natural hormones)?

A. We cannot make specific recommendations about other hormone medications, such as different estrogens or progestins. We also cannot make recommendations about hormones women take in lower dosages or in different ways, such as patches instead of pills.

Further, without scientific clinical trial data, one cannot assume that alternative estrogen plus progestin treatments are any safer than those studied in WHI.

Q. I am taking prescription hormones, what should I do?

A. We recommend that you talk with your health care provider about your individual health risk profile and the hormones you are currently taking.

Q. Does this new information apply to Selective Estrogen Receptor Modulators (SERMS) or phyto-estrogens?

A. These preparations were not studied in the WHI Hormone Program, and therefore, we cannot make any conclusions about the risks or benefits of SERMs, such as raloxifene (Evista®) or tamoxifen (Nolvadex®®) or phyto-estrogens.

Q. How does all of this new information affect my decision to use HRT for relief from hot flashes, sleep problems and mood swings?

A. The WHI and the observational studies on the risk of ovarian cancer were long-term studies which were not meant to address the shorter-term use of HRT. Thus, the information from these studies should be used by women considering use of HRT for longer than 3 or 4 years.

NATIONAL CANCER INSTITUTE

News from the NCI

UPDATED: July 16, 2002

Questions and Answers: Use of Hormones After Menopause

1. What is menopause?

Menopause is the transition between a woman's childbearing years and her non-childbearing years. It is the last stage of a biological process during which the ovaries gradually produce lower levels of sex hormones - estrogen, progesterone, and testosterone. By the time natural menopause is complete (usually between ages 45 and 55), hormone output decreases significantly. Women who have surgery to remove both of their ovaries (an operation called bilateral oophorectomy) experience "surgical menopause," the immediate cessation of ovarian hormone production and menstruation.

In postmenopausal women, estrogen levels are about one-tenth the level in premenopausal women and progesterone is nearly absent. The low levels of estrogen after menopause are produced by the adrenal glands and fat cells. Estrogen usage, with or without progestin, approximately doubles the estrogen level of a postmenopausal woman. Therefore, even with hormone treatment, estrogen and progesterone levels of a postmenopausal woman do not reach the natural levels of a premenopausal woman.

2. What hormones may be used after menopause?

Postmenopausal hormone use usually involves treatment with either estrogen alone or in combination with progestin to compensate for the decrease in natural hormones that occurs at menopause.

Estrogen is a natural hormone manufactured primarily by the ovaries. It is involved in the development and maintenance of secondary sex characteristics such as breasts in females and affects many aspects of women's physical and emotional health. Progestins are preparations that have effects similar to those of the natural hormone progesterone, which is primarily responsible for regulating the reproductive cycle. Among women who use postmenopausal hormones, women who have had their uterus removed use estrogen alone, whereas women with a uterus take a combination of estrogen plus progestin.

About 8 million women in the United States take estrogen alone and about 6 million women are on the combined hormone regimen, according to drug company estimates. Data from a national survey showed that 45 percent of U.S. women born between 1897 and 1950 used postmenopausal hormones for at least one month and 20 percent continued use for five or more years (1).

3. Why are hormones used after menopause?

Doctors may recommend using estrogen alone (if a woman does not have a uterus) or in combination with progestin to counter some of the possible effects of natural or surgical menopause on a woman's health and quality of life. Symptoms of menopause may include hot flashes, night sweats, sleeplessness, and vaginal dryness.

Hormones have also traditionally been prescribed to prevent some long-term conditions that are more common in women after menopause, such as osteoporosis and coronary heart disease (CHD). However, recent results from the Women's Health Initiative (WHI), a large randomized trial sponsored by the National Institutes of Health (NIH), have shown that overall, the risks of long-term estrogen with progestin outweigh the benefits. According to these results, estrogen with progestin increases the risk of both cardiovascular disease and breast cancer. Women should discuss risks and benefits of combined hormone use with their health care provider before selecting hormones for use in preventing osteoporosis (2). The results for use of estrogen alone are not yet known.

4. What are the effects of postmenopausal hormone use on the uterus?

Studies have shown that prolonged exposure of the uterus to estrogen without progesterone increases a women's risk of endometrial cancer (cancer of the uterine lining). By adding progestin to the estrogen regimen, the risk of endometrial cancer can be reduced to nearly the same level as women not using estrogen (3). However, some studies have shown increases in endometrial cancer risk with the combined regimens if progestins are used for less than ten days per month (4, 5).

Generally, standard postmenopausal hormones for women who have undergone hysterectomy (surgical removal of uterus) has been estrogen alone, whereas women who have not undergone this procedure have been given the estrogen-progestin combination.

5. What is known about the effects of postmenopausal hormones on heart disease?

The estrogen and progestin component of the Women's Health Initiative, which included over 16,000 women, compared two groups of healthy women (no prior history of heart disease), one using estrogen with progestin and one taking a placebo. In this study, combined estrogen and progestin was associated with a 22 percent increased risk of cardiovascular disease. The incidence of heart attacks increased 29 percent among women taking estrogen and progestin, as compared to the group of women on placebo (2). These effects became apparent after an average of 5.2 years of follow-up.

Another randomized trial, the Heart and Estrogen/progestin Replacement Study, recently concluded that estrogen in combination with progestin has no beneficial effects on the heart. Although earlier results from this study had suggested such benefits might exist, longer follow-up (6.8 years) found no overall reduction in the risk of heart attacks and coronary deaths with use of estrogen and progestin (6).

Some observational studies in which women reported whether they had used postmenopausal hormones have found evidence of a protective effect against CHD with use of estrogen alone (7). Most of the participants in these studies were healthy women at low risk for CHD. The WHI is continuing to investigate the potential benefits and risks of estrogen therapy on the heart in a randomized clinical trial that is expected to conclude in 2005.

6. What is known about the effects of postmenopausal hormones on bone health?

Postmenopausal osteoporosis is characterized by decreased bone mass, deterioration of bone tissue, and increased bone fragility, making bone fractures of great concern. Low levels of estrogen are a risk factor for osteoporosis in women.

Estrogen alone and estrogen combined with progestin have been shown to protect against osteoporosis. Definitive data from a recent large clinical trial support the ability of estrogen with progestin to prevent fractures at the hip, vertebrae, and other sites (2). However, some studies have shown that the beneficial effects of short-term therapy are not permanent; short-term use (three to five years) of estrogen to relieve symptoms of menopause did very little to prevent fractures from osteoporosis in women when they reached ages 75 to 80 years old (8, 9). Women who take estrogen to maintain bone density must continue taking estrogen because its beneficial effects on bone health disappear after hormone use is discontinued.

7. How does postmenopausal hormone use affect breast cancer risk and survival?

The estrogen and progestin component of the Women's Health Initiative concluded definitively in 2002 that combined estrogen and progestin therapy increases the risk of invasive breast cancer. After an average of five years of follow-up for each of more than 16,000 women in the study, the study found a 26 percent increase in breast cancer risk as compared to women taking placebo (2).

After five years of follow-up, the WHI study had found no indication of an increased incidence of breast cancer in the group of 11,000 trial participants taking estrogen alone (2). This clinical trial of estrogen vs. placebo is continuing. Observational studies, however, do indicate an increase in risk among women taking estrogen alone. A recent re-analysis of over 90 percent of breast cancer studies throughout the world showed an increased risk in breast cancer for women who used postmenopausal hormones for five years or longer. Most of the women included in this re-analysis were on estrogen alone. In this study, the increase in risk was seen not only in current users, but also in women who stopped therapy some time in the previous four years. No increased risk was seen in women who had stopped therapy more than four years earlier (10).

While observational studies indicate that both groups of hormone users have a higher risk of breast cancer than non-users, the risk appears to be greater among women using combined therapy than in women using estrogen alone (11, 12). One recent observational study found that risk increased with longer duration of hormone use and returned to the risk of non-users five or more years after use was stopped (12).

For women diagnosed with breast cancer, previous use of estrogen alone may have survival benefits. One study of breast cancer patients showed that users of estrogen had lower mortality rates from breast cancer than non-users. Most of these patients stopped using estrogen at the time of diagnosis. However, this protective effect diminished with time (15).

8. Is there a risk of ovarian cancer associated with postmenopausal hormone use?

A recent study that followed 44,241 postmenopausal women for approximately 20 years concluded that estrogen use is associated with an increased risk of ovarian cancer. In this study, women who used estrogen alone for 10-19 years were twice as likely to develop ovarian cancer than women who did not use postmenopausal hormones. For women who used estrogen for 20 or more years, the risk of ovarian cancer increased to three times that of women who did not use postmenopausal hormones (Lacey). Another recent large study also found an association between estrogen use and death due to ovarian cancer. In this study, the increased risk appeared to be limited to women who used estrogens for 10 or more years (16).

Because most studies have followed women using estrogen alone, there are currently not enough data to assess the potential effects of the estrogen-progestin combination on ovarian cancer (14). The above study of 44,241 postmenopausal women found that those who used estrogen in combination with progestin were not at increased risk of ovarian cancer, but the number of women in the study that had used estrogen plus progestin was small. More data are needed to determine whether estrogen-progestin has any effect on ovarian cancer risk (Lacey). One recent study suggested that combined estrogen-progestin regimens do not increase the risk of ovarian cancer if progestin is used for more than 15 days per month (15). More research is needed to clarify the relationship between postmenopausal hormone use and the risk of ovarian cancer in postmenopausal women.

9. What are the mortality benefits associated with postmenopausal hormone use?

Studies have shown a slightly lower total mortality rate among postmenopausal women using hormones. However, the WHI trial of estrogen plus progestin found no change in overall mortality associated with hormone use (2).

10. Are there other reported benefits or risks associated with postmenopausal hormone use?

Estrogen is very effective for treating menopausal symptoms such as hot flashes, sleeplessness, and vaginal dryness. Estrogen does not appear to be an effective treatment for these symptoms when they occur in older women (18).

Postmenopausal hormones may improve mood and psychological well-being in women who have hot flashes and sleeplessness during menopause, but should not be used to treat the symptoms of major depression. There are other reports that estrogen prevents memory loss, delays the onset of Alzheimer's disease, and improves urinary incontinence. However, there are no convincing clinical trial data to support these claims (19).

After five years of follow-up of women taking combined therapy, the Women's Health Initiative reported a 37 percent reduction in colorectal cancer cases compared to women on placebo. Further studies will be needed to confirm this finding (2).

Women who use estrogen plus progestin are at increased risk for blood clots (20, 21), gallbladder disease (21, 22, 23), and stroke (2, 24). Increased cases of blood clots in the lung (pulmonary embolisms) and inflammation of veins (thrombophlebitis) have also been reported with hormone use (25).

11. What are the risks of postmenopausal hormones for women who have a previous cancer history?

One of estrogen's primary roles is to promote the growth of cells in the breast and uterus. For this reason, there is concern that use of postmenopausal estrogen after cancer may promote further tumor growth. However, the safety of replacing women's estrogens after endometrial and breast cancer remains uncertain (26).

Only a small amount of research has been done to look at the risks associated with postmenopausal hormones for women who have a history of endometrial cancer. A few small studies have found no evidence that hormone use adversely influences survival and/or recurrence of the disease in these women (27). However, there have been no large, long-term studies to compare the potential benefits (protection against bone loss and heart disease) to the potential cancer risks. An ongoing study (Estrogen Replacement Therapy Study) sponsored by the National Cancer Institute is designed to resolve the debate over whether women who have had early-stage cancer of the uterus, or endometrial cancer, can safely take estrogen replacement therapy.

One study of breast cancer patients reported no increase in recurrence or mortality among women who continued hormone use following their diagnosis (28). Most of the women in this study were using estrogen alone.

12. Does the route of administration of hormones make a difference?

Most of the data on the long-term health effects of hormones come from studies involving estrogen and/or progestin pills. Other routes of administration of hormones are available, such as transdermal patches, estrogen gels, and vaginal creams and rings. These forms of estrogen are all equally effective methods of treating the symptoms of menopause, such as hot flashes and vaginal dryness.

There is also evidence to suggest that transdermal estrogen patches have beneficial effects on blood lipids, cholesterol, and bone, although many of these benefits are reduced as compared to hormones administered orally. Several studies have found the benefit of transdermal products on bone density and bone metabolism to be comparable to that of oral therapy (29, 30, 31).

The amount of estrogen that enters the blood stream from estrogen-containing vaginal creams and rings depends on the types of hormones and the dose. Generally, vaginal administration of hormones will result in lower levels of circulating hormones compared to an equivalent oral dose. Because the vaginal epithelium will respond to very small doses of estrogen, low-dose estrogen-containing creams can be used to correct vaginal atrophy. Vaginal estrogen therapy does not appear to protect against bone loss or cardiovascular disease (29, 30).

13. Are there any alternatives for women who choose not to take postmenopausal hormones?

Although postmenopausal hormones can have short-term beneficial effects, there are several health concerns associated with it, and many women may not feel that hormones are a good choice for them. Women should discuss with their health care provider whether to take postmenopausal hormones and what alternatives may be appropriate for them.

All women can adopt a healthy lifestyle, such as not smoking, regular exercise, and good nutrition (32). In addition, other prescription drugs, such as statins or beta-blockers, are available to lower blood lipid levels or blood pressure levels (33).

A healthy lifestyle can also help decrease a woman's risk of bone loss. In addition, health professionals also recommend calcium and vitamin D supplements as a means of preventing osteoporosis (34). Other drugs, such as Raloxifene®, Tibolone®, Alendronate®, and Risedronate® have been shown to prevent bone loss. These drugs increasingly are becoming the treatment of choice for osteoporosis in many postmenopausal women. (35). The investigational drug PTH (parathyroid hormone) is another prevention approach being evaluated in clinical trials.

Many women find relief from short-term menopause-related changes with non-prescription remedies, such as estrogen-containing foods (soy products, whole-grain cereal, seeds, certain fruits and vegetables) and creams, certain herbs such as black cohosh, and vitamin E and vitamin B complexes. Researchers are studying the safety and efficacy of these therapies (34). Local non-hormonal therapy is available for vaginal dryness and urinary bladder conditions.

Short-term menopause-related changes may resolve on their own and frequently require no therapy at all.

14. What research still needs to be done?

Several studies are under way to help women make a more educated and informed choice about whether postmenopausal hormones are right for them. In particular, the risk-benefit ratio of estrogen alone for women who have had a hysterectomy is still being evaluated.

The Women's Health Initiative (2) focuses on strategies for preventing heart disease, breast and colorectal cancer, and osteoporosis in postmenopausal women (36). While the component of the study focusing on the effects of estrogens combined with progestins has closed, another part of WHI with 11,000 participants is focusing on the effect of estrogen alone on heart disease and osteoporosis and is expected to continue until 2005. The impact of estrogen alone on breast cancer risk will also be assessed.

Other parts of the WHI will evaluate the effect of a diet low in fats and high in fruits, vegetables, and grains on the prevention of breast cancer, colorectal cancer, and heart disease, as well as the effect of calcium and vitamin D supplements on the prevention of osteoporosis-related fractures.

M.E. Comments:

The NIH presents excellent questions and answers with regard to synthetic hormones and menopausal symptoms. However, how is it possible that Natural Progesterone Cream does not get even one mention? The main value of the WHI study is that it points out that Prempro™ should not be used for anything except menopausal symptoms. However, for menopausal symptoms there are far safer bio-identical natural hormones that do not increase the risk of breast cancer, cardiovascular disease, stroke, etc. Sometimes the best finding of a study is "Don't use the Treatment - Primum Non Nocere!" (Above All Do No Harm).

References

(1) Brett KM, Madans JH. Use of postmenopausal hormone replacement therapy: estimates from a nationally representative cohort study. *Am J Epidemiology* 1997; 145(6):536-45.

(2) Writing Group for the Women's Health Initiative. Risks and benefits of combined estrogen and progestin in healthy postmenopausal women: Principal results from the Women's Health Initiative randomized controlled trial. *JAMA-EXPRESS* 2002 .

(3) Tavani A, La Vecchia C. The adverse effects of hormone replacement therapy. *Drugs Aging* 1999;14(5):347-57.

(4) Pike MC, Peters RK, Cozen W, et al. Estrogen-progestin replacement therapy and endometrial cancer. *J Natl Cancer Inst* 1997;89:1110-1116.

(5) Beresford S, Weiss N, Voigt L, et al. Risk of endometrial cancer in relation to use of oestrogen combined with cyclic progestagen therapy in postmenopausal women. *Lancet* 1997;349:458-461.

(6) Grady D, Herrington D, Bittner V, Blumenthal R, Davidson M, Hlatky M, Hsia J, Hulley S, Herd A, Khan S, Newby LK, Waters D, Vittinghoff E, Wenger N. Cardiovascular disease outcomes during 6.8 years of hormone therapy. *JAMA* 2002; 288:49-57.

(7) Rosano GM, Painina G. Cardiovascular pharmacology of hormone replacement therapy. *Drugs Aging* 1999;15(3):219-234.

(8) Reid IR. Pharmacological management of osteoporosis in postmenopausal women: a comparative review. *Drugs Aging* 1999;15(5):349-63.

(9) Rosenberg S, Vandromme J, Ayata NB, et al. Osteoporosis Management. *Int J Fertil Womens Med* 1999;44(5):241-9.

(10) Collaborative Group on Hormonal Factors in Breast Cancer. Breast cancer and hormone replacement therapy. *Lancet* 1997;350:1047-1059.

(11) Ross RK, Paganini-Hill A, Wan PC, et al. Effective hormone replacement therapy on breast cancer risk: estrogen versus estrogen plus progestin. *J Natl Cancer Inst* 2000;92:328-332.

(12) Schairer C, Lubin J, Troisi R, et al. Menopausal estrogen and estrogen-progestin replacement therapy and breast cancer risk. *JAMA* 2000;283(4):485-491.

(13) Schairer C, Gail M, Byrne C, Rosenberg P, Sturgeon S, Brinton L, Hoover R. Estrogen replacement therapy and breast cancer survival in a large screening study. *J Natl Cancer Inst,* 1999;91:264-70.

(14) Lacey JV, Mink PJ, Lubin JH, Sherman ME, Troisi R, Hartge P, Schatzkin A, Schairer C. Menopausal hormone replacement therapy and risk of ovarian cancer in a prospective study. *JAMA* 2002.

(15) Rodriguez C, Patel AV, Calle EE, Jacob EJ, Thun MJ. Estrogen replacement therapy and ovarian cancer mortality in a large prospective study of US women. *JAMA* 2001;285:14

(16) Weiss NS, Rossing MA. Oestrogen-replacement therapy and risk of ovarian cancer. *Lancet* 2001;358:438.

(17) Riman T, Dickman PW, Nilsson S, Correria N, Nordlinder H, Magnusson CM, Weiderpass E, Persson I. Hormone replacement therapy and the risk of invasive ovarian cancer in Swedish women. *J Natl Cancer Inst* 2002;94:497-504.

(18) Hlatky MA, Boothroyd D, Vittinghoff E, Sharp P, Whooley MA, Heary and Estrogen/Progestin Replacement Study Research Group. Quality-of-life and depressive symptoms in postmenopausal women after receiving hormone therapy: results from the Heart and Estrogen/Progestin Replacement Study trial. *JAMA* 2002;287:591-596.

(19) International Position Paper on Women's Health and Menopause: A Comprehensive Approach. *Best Clinical Practices.*2002;Chapter 13.

(20) Grady D, Wenger NK, Herrington D, Khan S, Furberg C, Hunninhake D, Vittinghoff E, Hulley S. Postmenopausal hormone therapy increases risk for venous thromboembolic disease. The Heart and Estrogen/progestin Replacement Study. *Ann Intern Med* 2000;132:689-696.

(21) Hulley S, Furberg C, Barrett-Connor E, Cauley J, Grady D, Haskell W, Knopp R, Lowery M, Satterfield S, Schrott H, Vittinghoff E, Hunninghake D. Non-cardiovascular disease outcomes during 6.8 years of hormone therapy. *JAMA*. 2002; 288:58-66.

(22) Simon JA, Hunninghake DB, Agarwal SK, Cauley JA, Ireland CC, Pickar JH. Effect of estrogen plus progestin on risk for biliary tract surgery in postmenopausal women with coronary artery disease. The Heart and Estrogen/progestin Replacement Study. *Ann Intern Med* 2001;135:493-501.

(23) Katar F, Weiss NS, Strite SA. Noncontraceptive estrogen use and risk of gallstone disease in women. *Am J Public Health* 1988;78:564.

(24) Hulley S, Grady D, Bush T, et al. Randomized trial of estrogen plus progestin for secondary prevention of coronary heart disease in postmenopausal women. *JAMA* 1998;280(7):605-613.

(25) Castellsague J, Perez Gutthann S, Garcia Rodriguez LA. Recent epidemiological studies of the association between hormone replacement therapy and venous thromboembolism. A review. *Drug Safety* 1998;18(2):117-23.

(26) Seifert M, Galid A, Kubista E. Estrogen replacement therapy in women with a history of breast cancer. *Maturitas* 1999;32(2):63-8.

(27) Burger CW, van Leeuwin FE, Scala F, Cognomens P. Hormone replacement therapy in women treated for gynecological malignancy. *Maturates* 1999;32(2):69-76.

(28) AMARA ES, Rossing MA, Daqing JR, Almeria JG, Barrow WE, Weiss NS. Hormone replacement therapy after a diagnosis of breast cancer in relation to recurrence and mortality. *J Natl Cancer Inst* 2001;93:754-62.

(29) Baker V. Alternatives to oral estrogen replacement. *Obstet Gynecol Clin North Am* 1994;21(2):271-97.

(30) Sturdee DW. Current hormone replacement therapy: what are the shortcomings? Advances in delivery. *Int J Clin Pract* 1999;53(6):468-472.

(31) Ansbacher R. The pharmokinetics and efficacy of different estrogens are not equivalent. *Am J Obstet Gynecol* 2001;184:255-263.

(32) Mosca, L, Grundy SM, Judelson D, King K, Limacher M, Oparil S, Pasternak R, Pearson TA, Redberg RF, Smith SC, Winston M, Zinberg S. Guide to preventive cardiology for women. *Circulation* 1999;99:2480-2484.

(33) Seed M, Sands RH, McLaren M, Kirk G, Darko D. The effect of hormone replacement therapy and route of administration on selected cardiovascular risk factors in post-menopausal women. *Fam Pract* 2000;17:497-507.

(34) Keller C, Fullerton J, Mobley C. Supplemental and complementary alternatives to hormone replacement therapy. *Amer Acac Nurse Pract* 1999;11(5):187-98.

(35) Raloxifene approval ushers in new drug class for osteoporosis. Estrogen-receptor effects vary by tissue type. *Am J Health Syst Pharm* 1998;55(2):104.

(36) The Women's Health Initiative Study Group. Design of the Women's Health Initiative clinical trial and observational study. *Control Clin Trials* 1998;19(1):61-109.

ADDITIONAL REFERENCES

Brekwoldt M, Keck C, Karck U. Benefits and risks of hormone replacement therapy (HRT). *J Steroid Biochem Mol Bio* 1995;53(1-6):205-8.

Brinton LA, Schairer C. Postmenopausal hormone-replacement therapy: time for reappraisal? *N Engl J Med* 1997;336(25):1821-1822.

Bush TL, Whiteman MK. Hormone replacement therapy and risk of breast cancer. Editorial. *JAMA* 1999;281(22):2140-2141.

Oates MB, McGhan WF, Smith MD. Hormone replacement therapy: a review of the risk versus benefit-Part II. *Med Interface* 1997;10(1):108-14.

Colditz G, Rosner B, for the Nurses' Health Study Research Group. Use of estrogen plus progestin is associated with greater increase in breast cancer risk than estrogen alone. *Am J Epidemiol* 1998;147(suppl):84S.

Persson I, Weiderpass E, Bergvist L, et al. Risks of breast and endometrial cancer after estrogen and estrogen-progestin replacement. *Cancer Causes Control* 1999;10(4):253-260.

###

For more information about cancer, visit NCI's Web site for patients, public, and the mass media at http://www.cancer.gov

M.E. COMMENTS:

If the results would have shown that synthetic HRT reduced breast cancer, strokes, clots and heart disease, would doctors have questioned the study?? How many more studies do we need before doctors stop prescribing synthetic HRT??? Many doctors interviewed after the publication of the Women's Health Initiative study in the July 17, 2002 issue of the Journal of the American Medical Association, said that the results were exaggerated and women should not stop taking synthetic HRT.

ଔଓଔଓ

In the July 30, 2002 issue of the *Wall Street Journal* columnist Tara Parker-Pope writes ...

> ...much of the recent debate about hormone replacement therapy has been about whether women should stop taking hormones altogether. **But the reality is that most women, and their doctors, aren't likely to abandon prescription hormone drugs... for them, the big question now is which brand to choose.**

ଔଓଔଓ

In the November 2002 issue of *Chicago Life* a supplement to the *New York Times* medical writer Suzanne Boothby writes that ...

> ...**Dr. Bill Creasman, a professor of obstetrics and gynecology at the Medical University of South Carolina, says this data is really not new and that women who are on HRT should not be alarmed.**
>
> "The safety data monitoring board pulled the plug on it (the study) because there was an increased number of breast cancers." Creasman says. "Well, if you take a look at the data, there did appear to be an increased number of breast cancers but it was not statistically significant. In other words, that could have been due to chance by itself."

In an article in *"eFamily Practice News"* (September 1, 2002) contributing writer Kate Johnson writes "Controversy notwithstanding - Immediate Change in HRT Regimen Is Not Necessary"

> **Postmenopausal women on hormone replacement therapy should be reassured that they don't need to immediately stop treatment in light of the results of the Women's Health Initiative, according to Dr. Charles Hammond.**

"I don't want to see patients stampeding to cessation of treatments or to alternate treatments, which we know even less about, until there's been a national debate on what the study really means," Dr. Hammond, president of the American College of Obstetricians and Gynecologists, said in an interview during the annual Southern Obstetric and Gynecologic Seminar.

He stressed that this is his personal opinion and not necessarily that of the college. Dr. Hammond is an educational consultant to and/or a member of the speaker's panel for Wyeth-Ayerst Laboratories, Berlex Laboratories, and Solvay Pharmaceuticals.

..."It is too soon for us to give opinions and advice while we are facing this tidal wave of negativism from both the press and the public," he said.

..."My advice to patients is there's no urgency to make a change. Let's have a debate nationally and then decide what we as physicians are going to recommend and implement in the next months," said Dr. Hammond, professor of obstetrics and gynecology at Duke University in Durham, N.C.

Even if it does take several months for national organizations and medical societies to digest and interpret the results of the Women's Health Initiative, women who are continuing their HRT regimen during that time will not be putting themselves at undo risk, he said.

He added that many women have already decided to stop their HRT regimens even against the advice of their physicians. "I'm sure that's happening, and I wouldn't say it's dangerous. They may have bleeding if they have a uterus in place, and they may experience sleep disruption and hot flashes. It also creates the interesting issue that if indeed HRT causes an increase in heart problems in the first year, they may end up re-exposing themselves to the first year if they go off it and then back on again," he said.

M.E. Comments:

Synthetic HRT drugs are unavoidably dangerous. Are there any doctors who follow ***evidence based scientific medicine****, with respect to synthetic HRT, when it goes against their long held belief system?????*

CHAPTER V

NATURAL PROGESTERONE CREAM
FOR WOMEN

Scientific studies have shown that many of the following symptoms and conditions may be caused by hormonal imbalance because of excess estrogen ingestion and can be alleviated by the simple use of a totally safe transdermal natural progesterone cream applied twice daily for three to six months.

- breast tenderness
- cervical dysplasia
- decreased sex drive
- depression
- endometriosis
- fat gain - especially around the abdomen, hips & thighs
- fatigue
- fibrocystic breasts
- fibroids
- headaches
- hot flashes
- infertility
- insomnia
- irregular menstrual periods
- migraine headaches
- miscarriages
- mood swings
- night sweats
- osteoporosis
- PMS
- skin conditions (i.e. acne, seborrhea, rosaceae, psoriasis, keratosis)
- water retention
- vaginal dryness

The timing during your menstrual cycle and the amount of natural progesterone cream that you need to use to reduce EOS (estrogen overload syndrome) will depend and vary with the different symptoms that you are experiencing. Detailed information is available at www.homefirst.com or do a search on the web for natural progesterone cream.

WHY SO MUCH ESTROGEN?

The body regulates the production of estrogen and progesterone. However, we are exposed to so many extraneous sources of estrogen that the female endocrine system cannot maintain its hormone balance. Many young, middle aged and elderly women suffer from symptoms that are brought about by estrogen overload thus requiring supplemental progesterone to achieve hormone balance.

SOURCES OF ESTROGEN

1) Natural estrogen - produced by your body.
2) Synthetic estrogen (i.e. synthetic hormone replacement therapy, birth control pills). The pharmaceutical industry has developed a wide variety of synthetic estrogens, potentially more carcinogenic, which stay in the body longer than the natural estrogens. Ethanol estradiol is used in the birth control pills and is one example of a synthetic estrogen. Prolonged exposure to synthetic estrogen significantly increases the risk for developing breast cancer and EOS.
3) Xeno-estrogens, also known as pseudo-estrogens, are synthetic chemicals in products such as pesticides, plastic, solvents, adhesives, car exhaust, industrial waste (i.e. PCBs and dioxins) and in meat from livestock fed estrogenic drugs to fatten them up. These xeno-estrogens exert hormonal influences on all living creatures by disrupting reproductive abilities and hormonal balance. Several dietary contaminants,

industrial chemicals and insecticides mimic estrogen. Although chemically quite different from estrogen, they affect menstrual and reproductive cycles as well as triggering both normal and abnormal cell division.

4) Phyto-estrogens (plant derived). Certain plants contain substances that have estrogenic effects in the body. Some phyto-estrogens (i.e. soybeans, tofu), stimulate the production of estrogen; however, other phyto-estrogens such as zeranol, which is used to fatten cattle, and is found in certain fungi, can disrupt the body's balance of estrogen, placing one into EOS (estrogen overload syndrome) and producing all its potential problems.

Why Do Many Women Need Supplemental Progesterone?

All estrogens, without the balance of progesterone, will increase cell proliferation, can be a precursor or cause of cancer (breast, uterus, cervix, ovaries, etc.) and can cause EOS.

We are living in a sea of estrogen. From the birth control pill to hormone replacement therapy to synthetic chemicals to phyto-estrogens, we ingest estrogen from youth to grave. Environmental and food sources which contain high levels of estrogen-like compounds may cause symptoms of EOS, even if you never used the birth control pill or HRT. The use of a natural progesterone will curtail the cellular proliferation effects of estrogen.

WHY NATURAL PROGESTERONE??... *OR* WHY SYNTHETIC PROGESTERONE HAS NOT SOLVED THE PROBLEM OF EOS ?

About 50 years ago scientists discovered that the Mexican wild yam contains substances which are chemically similar to human progesterone. Through fermentation and other steps in the laboratory scientists converted this substance into a molecular structure **identical** to the progesterone produced by the human body.

Doctors have begun to recognize the potential problems of hormone imbalance. To solve this problem they have added synthetic progesterone to the birth control pill as well as to the hormone replacement therapy regimens. However, these synthetic progesterone hormones (i.e. Provera®, Depo-Provera®, progestins) are all poorly absorbed, do not have the effect of countering the effects of estrogen hormones and cause many serious side effects. These synthetic chemicals have been linked to many serious side-effects. A partial listing from the PDR [Physicians Desk Reference] includes high blood pressure, blood clots in the lung and brain, headaches, changes in libido, fatigue, hirsutism, hemorrhagic eruptions and coagulation problems. **Natural progesterones work without any of the serious side effects of the synthetic progesterones.** Products such as natural progesterone cannot be patented. The pharmaceutical companies, in order to patent their designer progestin products, must alter the natural progesterone.

What To Do

If you are taking the birth control pill **stop**. If you are taking synthetic hormone replacement therapy drugs (i.e. Premarin®, Provera®) see a physician who understands the concept of EOS and will help you with a natural program that will restore your hormonal balance. Natural progesterone cream can actually help achieve hormone balance. Natural progesterone cream is absorbed through the skin and can act to reverse many of the EOS symptoms. Natural progesterone cream is not altered by the liver to create other potentially harmful compounds.

Are All Natural Progesterone Creams The Same

Not all natural progesterone creams have the same amount of natural progesterone. The physiologic dose is approximately 30-40 mg. per day. The percentage of natural progesterone cream may be too low or too high. They range from as little as 100 mg. per ounce to 1,000 mg. per ounce. In order to reach the physiologic dose of 30-40 mg. per day, the amount of cream you would have to use would range from one-third of an ounce to one-thirtieth of an ounce.

Some products are actually wild yam extracts which may be progestin, a compound with progestational activity but not the equivalent of bio-identical human, progesterone. Be sure that the natural progesterone cream that you use falls into the proper category. Also, be aware some products will contain other ingredients which may hinder or alter absorption.

Questions & Answers

Q. Do I need to see a physician to be on a program of natural progesterone cream?

A. Yes, even though natural progesterone cream is not a prescription item, it is advisable to have a consultation with a physician who is well versed in the issue of natural vs. synthetic hormone treatment. That physician will be able to advise you on the proper application and dosage.

Q. Can my estrogen and progesterone levels be measured?

A. Yes, estrogen and progesterone levels can be measured.

Q. Is it necessary to test my hormone levels?

A. In most cases hormone balance can be achieved without measuring the levels. The disappearance of symptoms with the use of natural progesterone cream will tell you that your hormones are in balance even without knowing the specific levels.

Q. Is there a time limit on how long I can use natural progesterone cream?

A. No. However, if you become asymptomatic you may want to consult with your physician on the proper dosage.

Q. How long until I see results?

A. Results will vary, however, usually you will see some results within two to three weeks.

Q. I have been using natural progesterone cream for three months and I'm still having menopausal symptoms, i.e. hot flashes, night sweats, vaginal dryness, etc., what should I do?

A. Ninety percent of women will have relief of their symptoms with natural progesterone cream. The other ten percent will require other treatments. I recommend you find a healthcare professional who will help relieve your symptoms without the use of synthetic hormones.

Q. I have read on the internet that natural estriol cream is a safe bio-identical estrogen which can be used instead of synthetic estrogens.

A. The jury is still out with regard to natural estriol cream. It is bio-identical and there have been studies alleging that it does not have the endometrial proliferation effects of other estrogens. However, the National Toxicology Program has recommended that all estrogens, including estriol, be placed on the list of "Known Human Carcinogens". Dr. Ray Peat, one of the leading researchers to demonstrate the value of progesterone, has taken a position that estriol may be just as dangerous as the other estrogens. To find a link to Dr. Peat's work see the Homefirst® web page at www.homefirst.com.

Q. My doctor says that I have fibroids and should have a hysterectomy. Will natural progesterone cream help?

A. Many times fibroids are caused by EOS (estrogen overload syndrome) and will shrink with the use of natural progesterone cream.

Q. My doctor says that I have polycystic ovarian (PCOS) syndrome. Will natural progesterone cream help?

A. Many times PCOS prevents ovulation and thereby prevents the natural production of progesterone. Therefore, using natural progesterone cream helps to restore the proper hormonal balance.

Q. My physician says that I have endometriosis. Will natural progesterone cream help?

A. Endometriosis has many possible causes. If the cause is hormone imbalance, the natural progesterone cream will help.

Q. I have been diagnosed with PMS. Will natural progesterone cream help?

A. If the PMS is caused by hormone imbalance, natural progesterone cream will help.

Q. Before my period my breasts are lumpy and painful. What can I do?

A. This condition is known as fibrocystic breast disease. It is sometimes caused by hormone imbalance and can be helped with natural progesterone cream.

Q. I am experiencing hot flashes and my doctor told me I need estrogen to control these symptoms.

A. Many times progesterone will alleviate hot flashes without any side effects. Before trying a trial of estrogen, I would recommend natural progesterone cream.

Q. Can natural progesterone cream help with PMS, EOS (estrogen overload syndrome) endometriosis or fibrocystic breast disease?

A. Yes, because progesterone is the precursor hormone helping to normalize all other endocrine and hormonal activity in the body. It assists in lowering the level of estrogen in the body, thus helping to alleviate these diseases and achieve hormone balance. Research has shown that women with PMS, endometriosis, or fibrocystic breast disease tend to have lower progesterone levels and 90% of these women can be successfully treated with natural progesterone.

Q. Does natural progesterone cream help vaginal dryness?

A. Yes, natural hormones in a cream base can be used intra-vaginally and can be used in treating vaginal dryness and vulvar atrophy associated with aging.

Q. I am already taking *synthetic hormone replacement therapy (Premarin®, Provera®) from my doctor, can I switch to natural progesterone cream?*

A. Yes, you can. Most women simply need to lower their dose of estrogen and replace the progestin (the "pro" part of the PremPro™) with progesterone cream. If you stop PremPro™ abruptly you will likely have a return of menopausal symptoms. It is advisable, however, to consult with a physician familiar with natural progesterone treatment. Natural hormones are simply a safe alternative to hormone replacement therapy. Synthetic hormones have many side effects and can be dangerous to your health.

Q. When and where should the natural progesterone cream be applied?

A. Morning and night to areas of soft skin such as the face, hands, chest, breast, inner arms, soles of feet. Periodically apply to different areas of the skin. The cream is readily absorbed and leaves no trace after a few minutes.

Q. Are there any other benefits of natural progesterone cream use?

A. Additional benefits which have been reported include: improved brain function, improved sleep pattern, diminished muscular aches and pains, improvement of skin problems, including acne, seborrhea, rosaceae, psoriasis and keratosis.

Q. Will I experience any problems when I start using natural progesterone cream?

A. Most women will experience no side effects from natural progesterone. However, in some premenopausal women, the ones in estrogen overload, it is possible that the initial application of progesterone will cause water retention, headaches, and swollen breasts (estrogenic activity). This happens because even though estrogen and progesterone generally have opposite effects in a cell, if a woman is deficient in progesterone, the initial use of natural progesterone will temporarily enhance estrogenic activity. When estrogen and progesterone levels are in proper balance, the effects of estrogen are opposed and the breast tenderness and other symptoms go away. This should not be longer than two to three months.

Q. Can I use too much natural progesterone cream?

A. Yes, it contains an active hormone. Even though there are no known side effects from the use of natural progesterone cream, it is important to use the proper range of dosage. If you start to experience symptoms such as tiredness and lethargy, you are most probably using too much.

REFERENCES

Lee, M.D., John. What Your Doctor May Not Tell You About Menopause: The Breakthrough Book on Natural Progesterone, 1996.

Lee, M.D., John R., What Your Doctor May *Not* Tell You about PREMENOPAUSE, (Balancing Your Hormones and Your Life From Thirty to Fifty) Warner Books, 1999.

Women considering synthetic hormone replacement therapy (HRT) for menopause symptoms and health benefits should read this book first. Lee has studied the research and concludes that estrogen is not the magic bullet for protection against heart disease and osteoporosis, nor does it retard aging. Natural progesterone, instead, puts postmenopausal women's hormones in balance. Dr. Lee cites study after study that indicates that natural progesterone, obtained in cream form, delivers what the synthetic HRT only promises.

Lee, M.D., John. What Your Doctor May Not Tell You About Breast Cancer 2002.

Martin, Gerstung, The Estrogen Alternative: Natural Hormone Therapy With Botanical Progesterone, Healing Arts Press, 1998.

Wright, M.D., Jonathan, V. Natural Hormone Replacement For Women Over 45; Smart Publications, 1997.

www.homefirst.com Detailed information is presented regarding dosage and usage of natural progesterone cream. Also contains multiple links to other valuable sites with scientific information about natural progesterone cream.

APPENDIX A

THE BIRTH CONTROL "PILL"
UNAVOIDABLY DANGEROUS

"Choose Life"

Deuteronomy 30:19

No other drug in the Physician's Desk Reference has as long a description of side effects as the birth control "PILL." Breast cancer, cardiovascular disease, blood clots, liver tumors, high blood pressure, infertility, sterility, and abortion are some of the more serious problems associated with the "PILL." In fact, the new third generation "PILL" seems to be more dangerous than the previous ones. This is not surprising. The late Dr. Robert Mendelsohn said, "Doctors don't let go of one medication until they find a more dangerous and profitable one to replace it." The dangers of the "PILL" are well documented. Doctors believe that no woman should be deprived of her "PILL" (a form of chemical steroids) so they prescribe the "PILL" for a list of completely contra-indicated medical conditions such as: irregular periods, scanty periods, no periods, ovarian cysts and even acne. When asked about the side effects of the "PILL" most doctors will tell you, *"trust me, it's safer than being pregnant."* This thinking reflects most doctor's views that pregnancy is a disease for which the "PILL" is the cure. If you are a teenager don't take the "PILL"! If you are thinking about ever having children, don't take the "PILL"!! If you're not thinking of having children, don't take the "PILL"!!! The "PILL" is unavoidably dangerous. As a medical student in 1971, I met Dr. Herbert Ratner. This distinguished physician and mentor became one of the most inspiring people in my life. Not only did Dr. Ratner teach my wife, Karen, and I the importance of children and family, he also informed us of the medical risks and hazards of the "PILL."

It is with great pleasure that I present an editorial written by the late Dr. Herbert Ratner;

The Medical Hazards of the Birth Control Pill

"To withdraw a drug once on the market is considerably more difficult than to get a drug on the market. FDA originally approved The Pill (Enovid) as safe for marketing on the basis of studies on only 132 women who had taken The Pill consecutively for 12 or more months. (Morton Mintz, *By Prescription Only*, Houghton Mifflin Co, Boston, 1967, p. 271.) Since The Pill has been on the market, the number of deaths reported in association with The Pill has far exceeded this number. In fact, it is safe to say that The Pill is the most dangerous drug ever introduced for use by the healthy in respect to lethality and major complications.

To admit mistakes is not characteristic of the American scene. Governmental agencies are no exceptions. In addition, the pressures and manipulations by drug firms—and the people they subsidize—to prevent a drug from being removed from the market can be extraordinary.

This is especially true of The Pill. Everyone prefers to believe that The Pill is safe.

The net result of propaganda, which led to pronouncements of Pill safety out of so-called humanitarian considerations, was that thc real users of The Pill, the middle and upper classes of the U.S., were seduced away from well established and safe means of birth control.

Perhaps the most fallacious argument in defense of The Pill is that it prevents the hazards of pregnancy. How a Pill which places the woman in a continuous state of false pregnancy, which in turn reproduces the illnesses of occasional pregnancies, can be considered an advantage is beyond scientific comprehension. The English, in an attempt to water down their finding of 3 deaths per 100,000 women from thromboembolism by alleging that The Pill prevents 12 deaths per 100,000 from pregnancy, ignore two essential facts. The first is that the alternative to The Pill is not pregnancy, but other and safer means of conception control. The second is that prior poor health contributes to most of the deaths in pregnancy. Contrasting the death rate of healthy women on The Pill to healthy pregnant women results in an entirely different comparison.

In pregnancy, the vascular system of the body adjusts to accommodate a rapidly enlarging uterus. In false or Pill induced pseudopregnancy, the pelvic vascular system increases the blood supply, but there is no enlarging uterus to utilize the increase. This results in extensive pelvic venous congestion, a condition which causes distress to surgeons. Such unnatural congestion introduces a whole series of factors predisposing to thrombosis and embolic phenomena.

The second example relates to the hypercoaguable state of pregnancy. This state was described prior to the introduction of The Pill. (B. Alexander, M.D., et al, Increased Clotting Factors in Pregnancy, New England Journal of Medicine 256:10931097, Nov. 30, 1961.) "This (state) provides a means whereby rapid clotting may take place at the site of placental separation." (Louise L. Phillips, Ch. 12, "Modifications of the Coagulation Mechanism During Pregnancy," in Modern Trends in Human Reproductive Physiology, Ed. H. M. Carey, Butterworths, 1963.) The Pill duplicates the hypercoaguable state. Because it serves no function in false pregnancy, its only contribution is to make the "patient potentially more susceptible to intravascular thrombosis." (Ibid,) The Pill introduces the risk without compensatory advantage.

The third example relates to the well known protection that pregnancy or embryonic tissue confer against certain induced cancers. In the absence of fetal tissue this protection is not conferred. We cannot assume that using The Pill contraceptively, confers this fetal-maternal relationship to human beings.

It would seem that if we had any respect for nature's economics, subtleties and the ordering of health, and any humility with respect to our multiple ignorances of the fetal-maternal relationship, we would more readily recognize that a state of false pregnancy is pathologic.

The first committee appointed to study the question of thromboembolism, in relation to The Pill, was sponsored by the manufacturers of Enovid, not the government, and conducted by the American Medical Association. (Proceedings of a Conference: Thromboembolic Phenomena in Women, Sept. 10, 1962, Chicago) The latter has a well known bias in favor of the pharmaceutical industry. Within several hours of convening this meeting, before participants had an adequate opportunity to study and discuss the data presented at the meeting, the Chairman called for a vote that would, in effect, be a whitewash of The Pill.

He commented, ". . . so far there has not been a single shred of evidence that has been presented in any of these figures to suggest that it contributes to a greater incidence of this disease. . . Will everyone agree with that?" The Chairman ultimately got the vote he requested. That it was not unanimous is a tribute to Stanford Wessler, M.D. a leading authority on thrombosis, who with courage and perspicacity, was the single dissenting voice.

If, for reasons of its own, the FDA feels it cannot remove The Pill from the market on the same basis as other drugs, we would urge the FDA to appoint another committee. If the safety of the public is paramount, such a committee should be sympathetic to a long established principle of medicine - *Above All Do No Harm!*"

Physician's Desk Reference 2002 - Excerpt from patient package insert

The serious side effects of the pill occur very infrequently, especially if you are in good health and are young. However, you should know that the following medical conditions have been associated with or made worse by the pill:

1. Blood clots in the legs (thrombophlebitis), lungs (pulmonary embolism), stoppage or rupture of a blood vessel in the brain (stroke), blockage of blood vessels in the heart (heart attack or angina pectoris) or other organs of the body.
2. Liver tumors, which may rupture and cause severe bleeding. A possible but not definite association has been found with the pill and liver cancer. However, liver cancers are extremely rare. The chance of developing liver cancer from using the pill is thus even rarer.
3. High blood pressure, although blood pressure usually returns to normal when the pill is stopped.

Third Generation Oral Contraception and Venous Thromboembolism

In April 1997 the *British Medical Journal* reported...

> "The published evidence confirms the Committee on Safety of Medicine's concerns.
>
> All studies indicated a statistically significant doubling of the adjusted odds ratios for venous thromboembolism in patients taking third rather than second generation oral contraceptive pills. These results are consistent with those from the transnational study published in this

issue of the *British Medical Journal*. The increased risk cannot be explained by known or expected bias or confounding.

The first law of epidemiology is that if a causal effect is large enough, it will show up despite all the problems of performing, analyzing, and interpreting observational studies on real people.

The doubling of risk of venous thromboembolism in users of third generation pills is important when the baseline risk in users of the pill is already three times greater than in non-users. Some studies have reported a relative risk of venous thrombo-embolism of about nine for users of third generation pills compared to women using non-hormonal contraception."

ORAL CONTRACEPTIVES AND RISK FOR BREAST CANCER IN YOUNG WOMAN

The following is text of a press release from the British National Cancer Institute Press Office. The research was reported in the Journal of the National Cancer Institute.

"A new study headed by scientists at the National Cancer Institute (NCI) adds to the evidence that oral contraceptives increase the risk of breast cancer in women under age 35. - *CancerNet News UK* June 6, 1995

'While the findings are reason for caution, breast cancer is uncommon in this age group, and the pill appears to be responsible for only a minority of breast cancers in young women,' said NCI's Louise A. Brinton, Ph.D., lead researcher of the study."

ORAL CONTRACEPTIVE, BREAST CANCER AND RELATION TO FFTP (FIRST FULL TERM PREGNANCY)

Development of a woman's breast depends on the female sex hormones estradiol and progesterone. Normal development, (Figure 1), requires a proper balance of the two hormones. However, when the breast is exposed to synthetic estrogen and/or progestins before a FFTP, the breast may be at risk for cancerous development. Before a FFTP the terminal ducts of the breast are immature and have not developed into fully formed lobules (Figure 2). These terminal ducts contain many more immature or

Figure 1 - Normal Developed Breast

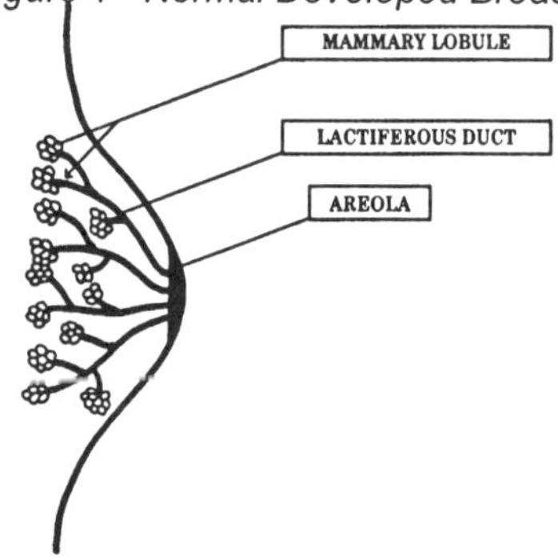

Figure 2 - Breast in Early Development

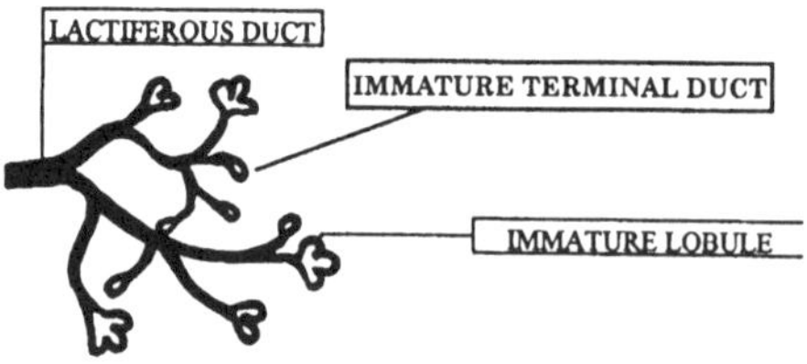

undifferentiated cells than are found in the mature lobule. The immature or undifferentiated cells are the most likely places where most breast cancer develops.

During pregnancy a woman's breasts are influenced by many hormones. The main three are estradiol, progesterone and hCG. These particular hormones reach levels that are far higher than those experienced by a woman at any other time of her life and cause a particularly rapid growth and maturation of the breast cells, especially during the first trimester of pregnancy. This is why women note breast tenderness and swelling during pregnancy. The combination of the high levels of estradiol, progesterone, and hCG during pregnancy serve to help complete the maturation process in the latter half of a woman's pregnancy.

After a woman delivers her first child, we see in Figure 3, that the breast has formed many mature lobules. These mature cells are more protected from carcinogenic (i.e. cancer producing) influence because many of them are fully differentiated (matured). Most cancers begin in immature terminal ducts in cells that are not fully differentiated.

Figure 3 - Fully Developed Breast

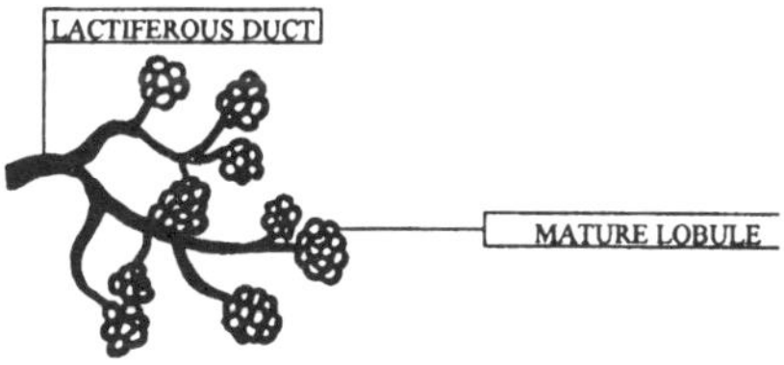

Several studies have suggested that the use of oral contraceptives in the early teen years may increase the risk of subsequent breast cancer.[1]

The largest meta-analysis done to date, a study that was published both in *The Lancet* and in *Contraception*, had no data on the risk of contraceptive use by women who use them prior to their FFTP. The latest meta-analysis which specifically examine the use of OCPs (oral contraceptive pills) to women who use them for four or more years prior to their FFTP was done by Dr. Isabelle Romieu in 1990.[2] Dr. Romieu noted that women who had taken OCPs for four or more years prior to their FFTP had a 72% increased risk of developing breast cancer.

M.E. COMMENTS:

I just recently became aware of the issue of OCPs used before FFTP. A full explanation is available in the outstanding book by Dr. Chris Kahlenborn, M.D. BREAST CANCER Its Link to Abortion and the Birth Control Pill.[3] The epidemic of breast cancer today may be directly related to the enormous number of women who not only are on the OCPs but who are taking them before a FFTP. If this research is further verified, it will become even more imperative to warn women of the increased risk of breast cancer when using OCPs before FFTP.

---

1. Haskell, CM. Cancer Treatment 4th ed. Philadelphia: WB Saunders Company; 1995.

2. Romier, I, Berlin, J, et al. Oral contraceptives and breast cancer, Review and meta-Analysis. Cancer 1990; 66: 2253-2263.

3. Kahlenborn, Chris M.D., BREAST CANCER, Its Link to Abortion and the Birth Control Pill One More Soul, 2000.

Sterility & INFERTILITY

Progress in Contraception Control: The Sequential Regimen. Physicians' Conference, San Francisco, April 4, 1965. Mead Johnson & Co., 1965.

> ". . . our multiparous patients . . . want to know how long it will be after they discontinue the tablets before they can expect to conceive... We have six patients who as yet have not become pregnant. They have been trying to conceive from two months up to thirty months. Because all have previously had children, we felt there must be some reason for the delay in conceiving." - *A. L. Banks, M.D. (University of Washington)*

> "I now have eight patients who are experiencing amenorrhea after discontinuing the combined contraceptive regimen . . . hoping to get pregnant. . ." - *Robert H. Hall, M.D. (University of Utah)*

> "Dr. Hall, you strike a very important chord in this discussion. I think Dr. Banks made reference to this point. All of us have encountered amenorrheic episodes following termination of the combined form of therapy." - *Robert B. Greenblatt, M.D. (Medical College of Georgia)*

ઉ෴ઉ෴

Amenorrhea After Treatment With Oral Contraceptives. R. P. Shearman M.D. (University of Sydney. Australia).

"In a period of 6 months, 9 women with secondary amenorrhea of at least 12 months duration, gave a history of onset after stopping The Pill." - *Lancet 2:1110-1111, Nov. 19, 1966.*

Syndrome of Anovulation Following Oral Contraceptives. O. I. Dodek, Jr., M.D. et al (Washington, D.C. Hospital Center).

"The anovulation syndrome is found in patients who have had amenorrhea or evidence of anovulation for three or more months after discontinuance of The Pill. Prolonged dysfunction of hypothalamic centers concerned with cyclic gonadotropin release is probably the cause." - *Am. J. Ob. and Gyn. 98 :1065-1070, 1967.*

Clomiphene Citrate for Improvement of Ovarian Function Georgeanna Seegar Jones, M.D. and Maria D. de Moraes-Ruehsen, M.D. (Johns Hopkins University).

"There were four women with longstanding amenorrhea (sterility) following oral contraception therapy." - *Am. J. Ob. & Gyn. 99:814-828, Nov. 15, 1967.*

Irregular Menses, Amenorrhea and Infertility Following Synthetic Progestational Agents. M. James Whitelaw, M.D. et al.

"During the past year we have had occasion to see 24 patients with normal menstrual cycles, but who, following the use of synthetic progestational agents (The Pill), had one or more of the following conditions as their chief complaint: irregular menses, amenorrhea, and infertility." Communication with other clinics indicates that there are hundreds of such cases that are unreported. "Let's Be Honest About The Pill" and inform nulliparous women, and those with only one living child of the possibility of being relatively infertile for undeterminate periods of time following discontinuation of oral contraceptives." - *JAMA 195:780-782, Feb. 28,1966.*

Should Nullipara and Infertility Patients be Given Oral Contraceptives? M. James Whitelaw, M.D. (Chief of Infertility Clinic, Santa Clara County Medical Center).

"Nullipara and infertility patients should not be given The Pill." - *New England Obstetrical and Gynecological Society, 39th Annual Meeting, Nov. 1, 1967.*

National Center for Health Statistics , 1988

In 1988 a panel assembled by the Congressional Office of Technology Assessment presented the following statistics to the U.S. Congress. Twenty five percent of couples in their thirties are infertile, even though only 1% of teenagers are infertile.

Wall Street Journal, 1993

Self-made Swiss billionaire, Fabio Bertarelli, whose company Serono Laboratories, manufactures 70 percent of the world's gonadotrophic hormones to treat infertility (including Pergonal and Metrodin), confirms this. In 1993 Bertarelli told the *Wall Street Journal,* "Our usual customers are women over 30 who have been taking birth-control pills since they were teenagers or in their early 20s."

ঙ্গ ঙ্গ

The Couples' Guide to Infertility, 1995

In the 1995 revised edition, Dr. Gary S. Berger and his associates again confirm the observations of Maggie Humm and Fabio Bertareli. "Long-term pill users may not menstruate or ovulate after they stop using the pill. This condition, known as post-pill amenorrhea, occurs because the pill disrupts the natural rhythmic flow of hormones from the hypothalamus to the pituitary to the ovaries. This may post a special problem for older women who have been on the pill for many years because their ovaries may have become resistant to resuming ovulation."

Cardiovascular Impact

Dr. Meir J. Stampfer in the *New England Journal of Medicine*, November 24, 1988 reported on the cardiovascular impacts of the birth control pill...

"The most dangerous and well-documented side effects commonly associated with the Pill are heart attacks and strokes. The eight-year Nurse's Health Study at Harvard Medical School found that Pill users are 250 percent as likely to have heart attacks and strokes than those who don't use the Pill, probably because the Pill excessively increases blood clotting ability.

However, one of the major findings of the study was that women who get off the Pill have rates of cardiovascular disease equal to that of the general population after a period of one year.

This study was based on an eight-year followup of 119,061 female nurses, ranging in age from 30 to 55 in 1980. 7,074 were current pill users and 49,269 were previous users. Overall, there was 380 heart attacks, 205 strokes, and 230 cardiovascular deaths among pill users."

UNAVOIDABLY UNSAFE

Thomas P. Monaghan, Co-Chairman, Free Speech Advocates wrote an article "Unavoidably Unsafe" in *Fidelity* Magazine, October 1987, pages 14 and 15...

"According to United States Federal Courts, the birth control pill has been

> classified as 'unavoidably unsafe.' This means that, implicit in a woman's consent to use the pill, even if she is not entirely informed of its dangers, is an acknowledgment of physical risk."

DISTURBING INFORMATION ON THE PILL

Dr. Ojvind Lidepaard, et al., Hvidovre University Clinic of Copenhagen, reporting in the *British Medical Journal* (April 1993 cited *Europe Today* No. 23, May 3, 1993) revealed that in a study of 2400 women aged 15 to 44, who were using the Birth control Pill, 800 suffered some degree of cerebral thrombosis. although not all of the blood clots led to stroke.

In the *Journal of American Medical Association*; Vol. 284 No. 14, October 11, 2000:1791-1798; *"Risk of Breast Cancer With Oral Contraceptive Use in Women With a Family History of Breast Cancer*" Grabrick, et al reports that...

> ...Oral Contraceptive (OC) use is weakly associated with breast cancer risk in the general population, but the association among women with a familial predisposition to breast cancer is less clear.

and concluded

> ...These results suggest that women who have ever used earlier formulations

> of Oral Contraceptives and who also have a first-degree relative with breast cancer may be at particularly high risk for breast cancer. Further studies of women with a strong family history who have used more recent lower-dosage formulations of Oral Contraceptives are needed to determine how women with a familial predisposition to breast cancer should be advised regarding Oral Contraceptive use today.

ଔଓଔଓ

In *British Medical Journal* BMJ 2001;323:131-134 (21 July 2001) "Third generation oral contraceptives and risk of venous thrombosis: meta-analysis" Kemmeren, et al. write...

> **Objective:** To evaluate quantitatively articles that compared effects of second and third generation oral contraceptives on risk of venous thrombosis.
>
> **...Discussion:** Our meta-analysis shows that third generation oral contraceptives are associated with a 1.7-fold increased risk of venous thrombosis compared with second generation oral contraceptives. After stratifying by various factors and examining selected subgroups, the increased risk remained.

and conclude...

> **Conclusion:** Our meta-analysis supports the view that third generation oral

> contraceptives are associated with a 1.7-fold increased risk of venous thrombosis compared with second generation oral contraceptives. The risk is highest in first time users. Although confounding can never be excluded with certainty in observational studies, it seems that the biases that have been suggested and examined are not sufficient to account for the results.

M.E. Comments:

Drug companies don't let go of one drug (second generation oral contraceptive pill until they find a more dangerous and profitable one to replace it (third generation oral contraceptive pill). Don't be fooled by drug companies and doctors trying to convince you that the newest treatments are better and safer. Many times the newer treatment turns out to be worse and even more dangerous.

In the *Archives of Internal Medicine*, Vol. 161 No. 16, September 10, 2001; 2000-2005, "Oral Contraceptive Use and Hormone Replacement Therapy Are Associated With Microalbuminuria" Monster, et al, reported...

> **Background:** Controversy exists regarding the adverse and beneficial effects of oral contraceptive use and hormone replacement therapy. Microalbuminuria is associated with

> increased risk of renal and cardiovascular disease.
>
> **...Conclusion:** Regular and long-term oral contraceptive use and hormone replacement therapy are associated with an increased risk for microalbuminuria and cardiovascular disease.

ଓଷଓଷ

In the *New England Journal of Medicine* Volume 345:1787-1793, December 20, 2001; Number 25, "Oral Contraceptives and the Risk of Myocardial Infarction" Tanis, et al., found...

> **Background:** An association between the use of oral contraceptives and the risk of myocardial infarction has been found in some, but not all, studies. We investigated this association, according to the type of progestagen included in third-generation (i.e., desogestrel or gestodene) and second-generation (i.e., levonorgestrel) oral contraceptives, the dose of estrogen, and the presence or absence of prothrombotic mutations.

and concluded...

> **Conclusions:** The risk of myocardial infarction was increased among women who used second-generation oral contraceptives. The results with respect to the use of third-generation oral contraceptives were inconclusive but

suggested that the risk was lower than the risk associated with second-generation oral contraceptives. The risk of myocardial infarction was similar among women who used oral contraceptives whether or not they had a prothrombotic mutation.

In *Contraception*, 61:1:2001; 51-58, "A Prospective Study of the Effects of Oral Contraceptives on Sexuality and Well-being and Their Relationship to Discontinuation, Sanders, et al., reported...

> ...Emotional and sexual side effects are the primary reason that reason discon-tinue or switch oral contraceptives. On regression analysis four variables explained 87% of the variance in outcome:
>
> emotional side effects, change in the frequency of sexual thoughts, effect on premenstrual symptoms, and decreased psychosexual arousability.

and recommended...

> Women should be encouraged to discuss sexual and emotion effects of oral contraceptives with their healthcare provider much the same way as they are encouraged to report physical effects such as bleeding, headaches, or breast tenderness.

M.E. Comments:

This study adds evidence to one of the effects of the oral contraceptive as altering sexual mood, just the opposite of what most women believe, i.e. that the birth control pill will allow them to be sexually uninhibited, but they find that they don't have the desire.

In *Lancet* Volume 359, Number 9312, 30 March 2002; 1085-1092, "Effect of oral contraceptives on risk of cervical cancer in women with human papillomavirus infection: the IARC multicentric case-control study", Moreno, et al. found...

> **Background: Use of oral contraceptives could increase risk of cervical cancer**; however, the effect of human papillomavirus (HPV), the main cause of cervical cancer, is not usually taken into account. We aimed to assess how use of oral contraceptives affected risk of cervical cancer in women who tested positive for HPV DNA.
>
> **Interpretation:** Long-term use of oral contraceptives could be a cofactor that increases risk of cervical carcinoma by up to four-fold in women who are positive for cervical HPV DNA. In the absence of worldwide information about HPV status, extra effort should be made to include long-term users of oral contraceptives in cervical screening programmes.

and in conclusion:

> **We think that our results lend support to the existence of an association between oral contraceptives and HPV**, and suggest that studies not restricted to women who were positive for HPV could have underestimated the effect of oral contraceptives. Our results could help

women who have persistent HPV infection to balance benefits (prevention of pregnancy and cancers of the ovary and corpus uteri) and harms of long-term oral contraceptive use, and suggest that long-term users of oral contraceptives should be included in cervical screening programmes.

ଓଃଓଃ

In *International Journal of Cancer 2002*; 101:427-433. "HPV infection linked to oncogene amplifications in cervical tumors." Wallin, M.D., et al. found...

Several oncogenes (genes which can potentially induce cancer transformation)are often amplified in cervical carcinomas associated with human papillomavirus (HPV) infection and concluded that...

...These findings indicate that HPV-associated cervical carcinomas bear frequent alterations of these genes, which may have critical biologic impact on the development and progression of carcinoma of the uterine cervix," the researchers conclude.

M.E. Comments

Add one more serious problem to the oral contraceptive pill, increased risk of human papillomavirus (HPV). HPV is a known risk factor for cervical cancer.

References

Berger, Dr. Gary S., The Couples' Guide to Infertility, 1995.

Couple to Couple League's website is http://www.ccli.org

Epstein, et al., The Breast Cancer Prevention Program, "Chapter 3, The Pill: Assessing Your Risks," Macmillan, U.S.A.

http://www.homefirst.com (The Homefirst® WEB page containing extensive links to research on the "Pill", as well as many related topics).

Mintz, Morton, The Pill An Alarming Report, (*Washington Post)* 1969.

Ratner, Herbert, M.D., "The Medical Hazards of the Birth Control Pill," Child and Family, 1970.

Seaman, Barbara, The Doctor's Case Against the Pill, 1995 (original publication 1969), Hunter House.

APPENDIX B

NATURAL PROGESTERONE CREAM
FOR MEN

MEN'S HORMONES

Progesterone and estradiol (an estrogen) are two hormones naturally produced by the male body, but in smaller amounts than in women and are vital to good health. Progesterone is the primary precursor of adrenal cortical hormones and testosterone. It also has the effect of balancing out the effects of estradiol. Uninhibited estradiol (estradiol without progesterone) has been implicated in prostate growth leading to BPH. As men age, their progesterone levels fall, causing their uninhibited estradiol levels to rise. It has been theorized that one of the causes of BPH may be inadequate amounts of progesterone synthesis needed to counteract the effect of estradiol.

BENIGN PROSTATIC HYPERTROPHY

(Non-Cancerous Enlargement of the Prostate)

The following are some of the symptoms that have been associated with BPH:

- straining to start a urinary stream
- a weak urinary stream
- dribbling of urine
- dysuria - painful urination
- incomplete emptying of bladder leading to cystitis
- discomfort during intercourse
- painful ejaculation
- impotence
- lowered sex drive
- the need to urinate frequently
- lower back pain

Somewhere between the ages of 30 and 40 a man's prostate begins to enlarge. The growth of the prostate is known as Benign Prostatic Hypertrophy (BPH). BPH will affect nearly all men as they age. What is generally not known is the fact that there are safe, natural and effective ways of dealing with BPH. By age 50 more than 50% of men will have prostate surgery, radiation treatment, or will be on prescription drugs like Proscar (finasteride). Finasteride has been shown to cause impotence in more than 60% of patients [*Physician's Desk Reference - PDR®*, Medical Economics, 2002], decreased libido, decreased amount of semen per ejaculation, breast tenderness, breast enlargement, lip swelling and skin rashes.

Scientific studies have shown that many of the symptoms of BPH may be alleviated by a combination of a natural progesterone cream applied twice a day, along with herbal vitamin and mineral pills which include some or all of the following: Saw Palmetto Berry (Serenoa Repens), Pygeum Africanum, American Ginseng (Panax Quinquefolius), Bearberry Extract (Arctostaphylos Uva-Ursi), Pumpkin Seed Oil, Vitamin C, Zinc, Lycopene, Vitamin B6, Magnesium, Stinging Nettle Leaves, Cernilton Flower Pollen, Flaxseed Oil, Evening Primrose Oil, Vitamin E, Copper, Amino Acids, Multi-vitamins and Minerals.

The main reason that men, who also have breasts and breast tissue, rarely develop breast cancer is that their exposure to estrogen is minimal. However, today men also have elevated estrogen levels because of unavoidable environmental and food sources which contain high levels of estrogen-like compounds. Xeno-estrogens, also known as pseudo-estrogens, are synthetic chemicals in products such as pesticides, plastics, solvents, adhesives, car exhaust, industrial waste (i.e. PCBs and dioxins), meat from livestock fed estrogenic drugs to fatten them up. These xeno-estrogens exert estrogen-like influences on all living creatures, male and female, by disrupting the reproductive abilities and hormonal balance. Several dietary contaminants, industrial chemicals and insecticides also act like estrogens.

Since uninhibited estrogen is one of the causes of enlargement of the prostate and symptoms of BPH, the role of progesterone is to balance this uninhibited estrogen. **In fact, natural progesterone may be the only remedy needed to reverse benign prostatic enlargement.** Men may also need progesterone to reverse the feminizing effects of too much estrogen.

WHY NATURAL PROGESTERONE ??

About 50 years ago scientists discovered that the Mexican wild yam contains substances which are chemically similar to human progesterone. Through fermentation and other steps in the laboratory scientists converted this substance into a molecular structure **identical** to the progesterone produced by the human body.

Products such as natural progesterone cannot be patented. The pharmaceutical companies, in order to patent their designer progestin products (now coming out for men), must alter natural progesterone. These altered chemicals have been linked to many serious side-effects (a partial listing from the PDR [Physicians Desk Reference] includes high blood pressure, blood clots in the lung and brain, headaches, changes in libido, fatigue, hemorrhagic eruptions, coagulation problems). **Natural progesterones work without any of the serious side effects of the altered synthetic progesterones and do not have any feminizing effect on men.**

Should You Try Alternatives to Surgery & Prescription Medication

Before beginning any hormone treatment, herbal treatment, vitamin treatment, etc. it is advisable to have a thorough medical evaluation to make sure that the genito-urinary problems are due to BPH and not due to infection, bladder stones, or cancer.

Natural Progesterone Cream

If the doctor determines your symptoms are caused by mild or moderate BPH, it is appropriate to consider natural options before proceeding to pharmaceutical agents or surgery. My recommendation is to begin with a natural progesterone cream, **as this may be the total solution to BPH.**

If you decide to use natural progesterone cream, it is important to use one that has the proper amount of natural progesterone. The amount of natural progesterone cream that you need to counteract the estrogenic effect and to cause the prostate to shrink, will depend and vary with the different symptoms that you are experiencing. The recommended physiologic dose for men is 8-12 mg. of progesterone daily.

The only side effect of natural progesterone cream for men, mentioned in the literature, is the potential for decreased sperm motility for men under the age of 35. This does not mean a decreased number of sperm; it means that your sperm do not move as quickly. Decreased motility can either be a positive or a negative depending on your desire for maximum fertility. There is no evidence that natural progesterone has any other side effects. Since BPH and its associated symptoms rarely start before age 40, this side effect will rarely be a significant factor.

SAW PALMETTO

Berries from the Saw Palmetto tree have been used to treat symptoms caused by the enlargement of the prostate gland, as far back as the Seminole Indians in Florida in the 1700s, according to the report in the November 10, 1998 issue of the Journal of the American Medical Association (*JAMA)*. In the *JAMA* study doctors reviewed 18 studies of Saw Palmetto use involving 2,939 patients with BPH. Men taking Saw Palmetto extract were nearly twice as likely to report improvements in symptoms than men taking placebos. When compared with Finasteride (Proscar®), a prescription drug to reduce the size of the prostate, Saw Palmetto provided similar relief without causing any of the side effects such as impotence. *(Urology* - 1998, Jun; 51(6): 1003-7) "Also, evidence suggests that Saw Palmetto improves urology symptoms and flow measures..." (*JAMA* 1998, Nov. 10; 280(18): 1604-9)

A similar study in the *Journal of Clinical Trials* concluded that Saw Palmetto is a well tolerated agent that may significantly improve lower urinary tract symptoms in men with BPH (*Urology* - 1998 Jun; 51(6): 1003-7).

LYCOPENE: A GOOD REASON TO EAT TOMATOES

Tomatoes contain numerous nutrients, among them: lycopene. A five year study of 48,000 men found that those eating 10 servings a week of cooked tomato products had the lowest risk of prostate cancer. Their risk was 1/3 that of men eating less than two servings per week. Other studies suggest that lycopene may play a role in reducing the risk of other cancers including colon and rectal cancers. (*Health Oasis Mayo Clinic* - 9/20/98) [http://www.mayohealth.org/mayo/9809/htm/tomato.htm]

ZINC

The ability to absorb zinc declines with age increasing the likelihood of developing BPH. A healthy prostate gland contains more zinc than any other organ in the body. Some experts believe that when zinc is needed in other parts of the body it is taken from the prostate, which is then left with a deficit of this trace mineral.

PHYTO MEDICINALS THAT SHOW PROMISE IN THE TREATMENT OF BPH

Pygeum Africanum and Pumpkin Seed Oil, are among the other phyto-medicinals that have shown promise in the treatment of BPH, without the serious side effects associated with Proscar, surgery, radiation or chemical drugs.

Questions and Answers

Q. Do I need to see a physician to be on a program of natural progesterone cream?

A. No, natural progesterone cream is not a prescription item. However, it is advisable to have a consultation with a physician who is well versed in the issue of natural vs. synthetic hormone treatment. That physician will be able to advise you on the proper application and dosage.

Q. Where should the natural progesterone cream be applied?

A. Morning and night to areas of soft skin such as the face, hands, chest, scrotum, inner arms, soles of feet. Periodically apply to different areas of the skin. The cream is readily absorbed and leaves no trace after a few minutes.

Q. Is natural progesterone cream for men a feminizing hormone?

A. No, that is the role of estrogen. Remember that in utero all babies (boys and girls) are exposed to high levels of progesterone.

Q. Do men produce progesterone?

A. Yes. The average man produces 8-12 mg. of progesterone per day.

Q. Can natural progesterone cream for men prevent or help BPH?

A. If the BPH is due to exposure to estrogen and estrogen-like compounds, the balancing effect of Natural progesterone cream for Men will shrink the prostate and reduce the symptoms.

Q. I get up five to six times a night to urinate. Will natural progesterone cream for men help?

A. If your frequent urination is related to BPH and if the BPH is from EOS natural progesterone cream for men may stop the frequent urination.

References for Prostate Health

Buck, A.C. "Phytotherapy for the Prostate." British Journal of Urology, 78:325-336, 1996.

Lowe, F.C. and J.C. Ku. "Phytotherapy in Treatment of Benign Prostatic Hyperplasia: A Critical Review," Urology 48(1):12-20, 1996.

"Lycopene - a good reason to eat tomatoes." Health Oasis Mayo Clinic, September 1998.

"Saw palmetto extracts for treatment of benign prostatic hyperplasia: a systematic review." JAMA 1998, Nov. 11; 280(18): 1604-9.

"Saw palmetto (Serenoa repens) in men with lower urinary tract symptoms: effects on urodynamic parameters and voiding symptoms." Urology - 1998, Jun; 51(6): 1003-7

www.homefirst.com - Detailed information is presented regarding dosage and usage of natural progesterone cream for men. Also contains multiple links to other valuable sites with scientific information about natural progesterone cream for men.

APPENDIX C

WYETH PHARMACEUTICALS LETTERS REGARDING PREMPRO™, PREMPHASE® AND PREMARIN®.

Following are two letters that I received from Wyeth regarding the Women's Health Initiative Study.

The first letter explains why the study was stopped and the second letter details some of the changes in the labeling of Prempro™, Premphase® and Premarin®. Even though the WIH study showed a decrease in fractures in the Prempro™ group, the recommendations were

> ...**When used solely for the prevention of postmenopausal osteoporosis, alternative treatments should be carefully considered.**

I find no indications for using the unavoidably dangerous Prempro™. For menopausal symptoms one should consult physicians who are familiar with alternatives, such as bio-identical natural progesterone cream.

Wyeth Pharmaceuticals
P.O. Box 8299
Philadelphia, PA 19101-8299

Wyeth®

July 2002

Dear Doctor:

We are writing to share with you important new information from the National Institutes of Health (NIH)-sponsored Women.s Health Initiative (WHI) clarifying the risks and benefits associated with combination hormone replacement therapy (HRT), whether provided in a single tablet or a 2-tablet combination of estrogen and progestin. These data will be of value to you in managing your menopausal patients who are currently using Prempro™ (conjugated estrogens/medroxyprogesterone acetate tablets, 0.625 mg /2.5 mg) or considering it, and especially those who are on or considering long-term therapy.

The WHI is a large-scale study of estrogen and combination estrogen plus progestin as preventive therapies for postmenopausal women, designed to assess the long-term risk/benefit ratio of estrogen replacement therapy (ERT) and combination HRT. It enrolled 27,000 women between 1993 and 1998 and is scheduled to conclude in 2005. A total of 16,608 women were randomized to combination HRT versus placebo.

The Data and Safety Monitoring Board (DSMB) of WHI has decided to discontinue the combination HRT arm of

RELATIVE AND ABSOLUTE RISK OR BENEFIT SEEN IN ESTROGEN PLUS PROGESTIN ARM OF WHI (n =16,608, placebo and study drug)			
Health Event	**Relative Risk vs. Placebo Group at 5.2 Years**	**Increased Absolute Risk per 10,000 Women/Year**	**Increased Absolute Benefit per 10,000 Women/Year**
Heart Attacks	1.29	7	
Strokes	1.41	8	
Breast Cancer	1.26	8	
Thromboembolic Events	2.11	18	
Colorectal Cancer	0.63		6
Hip Fractures	0.66		5

Adapted from *WHI HRT Update*, June 2002

the study, citing as the main factor an increased risk of invasive breast cancer in the group receiving continuous combined HRT compared to the placebo group after an average follow-up of 5.2 years. This, combined with an increase in cardiovascular events in women on active drug vs. those on placebo that began in the first year and persisted, outweighed the benefits, which included a reduced incidence of colon cancer and hip fractures.

Wyeth

Wyeth Pharmaceuticals
August 28, 2002

Important labeling update: new information to provide guidance in prescribing PREMPRO™/PREMPHASE® (conjugated estrogens/medroxyprogesterone acetate tablets) and PREMARIN® (conjugated estrogens tablets, USP)

Dear Health Care Professional:

We are writing to inform you of important new safety information in labeling regarding PREMPRO™ (conjugated estrogens/medroxyprogesterone acetate tablets), PREMPHASE® (conjugated estrogens/medroxyprogesterone acetate tablets), and PREMARIN® (conjugated estrogens tablets, USP). The labeling changes reflect new data, primarily from the Women's Health Initiative (WHI).

The new PREMPRO/PREMPHASE and PREMARIN labels provide additional information with regard to certain risks. Notably, several sections have been modified, including the INDICATIONS and USAGE, CONTRAINDICATIONS, WARNINGS, PRECAUTIONS, and DOSAGE and ADMINISTRATION sections. **Please be certain to read both entire labels (enclosed) carefully, as they include changes not reprinted in this letter.**

Please note that:

PREMPRO, PREMPHASE, and PREMARIN are not indicated and should not be used to prevent coronary heart disease.

The product indications remain the same. However, because of the potential increased risks of cardiovascular events, breast cancer and venous thromboembolic events, use of PREMPRO, PREMPHASE, and PREMARIN should be limited to the shortest duration consistent with treatment goals and risks for the individual woman, and should be periodically reevaluated. When used solely for the prevention of postmenopausal osteoporosis, alternative treatments should be carefully considered.

Wyeth will continue to work closely with the medical community and regulatory authorities to further refine its product labels for all of its postmenopausal hormone therapies, regardless of the estrogen or progestin used. We are dedicated to communicating new information to you and your patients. If you have additional questions, please call the PREMARIN® Family of Products information line at 1-800-842-1441.

Sincerely,

Victoria Kusiak

Victoria Kusiak, M.D.
Vice President, Global Medical Affairs and
North American Medical Director for Wyeth Pharmaceuticals

Index

About Homefirst®

Homefirst® Health Services provides a full range of services in family health care in the greater Chicago metropolitan area with eight medical centers - 847/679-8336 or www.homefirst.com. Our group of doctors, nurses, and certified nurse midwives dedicate themselves to providing the highest quality of health care standards while maintaining personalized care for each patient and family. We encourage patient involvement in the many decisions made regarding their health care.

Homefirst® provides a full range of obstetric and pediatric services, in addition to women's and men's health care. We continue to emphasize the philosophy of minimal use of drugs and surgery and maximal patient involvement in maintaining good health for everyone. We promote an integrative evidence based approach to managing illness. The majority of health problems are resolved by our medical staff. When necessary, we provide referrals to a wide variety of consultants which include practitioners in alternative approaches to medicine as well as conventional medical specialists.

The Homefirst® physicians have treated more than 3,000 women for pre- and post-menopausal symptoms. In keeping with our philosophy of minimal intervention we have found that over 90% of these women received relief with the safe alternative of natural progesterone cream.

It has been an honor and a privilege to serve families for over 30 years, to deliver more than 15,000 babies at home and serve over 75,000 mothers, fathers, children and extended family members. Our greatest pleasure has been to provide the opportunity for our patients to grow and enrich their lives with the knowledge they are taking charge over their own health and maximizing their greatest health potential.

About the Author
Dr. Mayer Eisenstein

Dr. Mayer Eisenstein is a graduate of the University of Illinois Medical School, the Medical College of Wisconsin School of Public Health, and the John Marshall Law School.

Since 1973 he has been in private medical practice and is currently the Medical Director of Homefirst® Health Services, the largest physician attended home birth service in the country. In his 30 years in medicine, he and his practice have delivered over 15,000 babies at home, as well as cared for over 75,000 parents, grandparents and children. Now, Dr. Eisenstein and his practice are delivering second generation babies for women who themselves were born at home with his practice.

He is Board Certified by the National Board of Medical Examiners, American Board of Public Health and Preventive Medicine, and the American Board of Quality Assurance and Utilization Review Physicians. He is a member of the National Honor Society. He is a recipient of the Howard Fellowship, Health Professional Scholarship, University of Illinois School of Medicine Scholarship, and is a member of the Illinois Bar.

He is on the Professional Board of the Family Life League, Council for the Jewish Elderly, Task Force Council on Education for Public Health - Medical College of Wisconsin, and on the Editorial Board for "Child and Family Magazine". He is the author of the award winning book *Give Birth at Home With The Home Birth Advantage*, *Safer Medicine, and Don't Vaccinate Before You Educate.* His medical film "Primum Non Nocere" (Above All Do No Harm), a documentary on home birth, was an award winner at the Chicago Film Festival in 1987.

Some of his guest appearances include: the "Phil Donahue Show", "Milt Rosenberg Show", "Today in Chicago", "Ask the Expert", "Daybreak", "Oprah Winfrey Show", "Ed Schwartz Radio Show". "WMAQ TV news 'Unnecessary Hysterectomy'", "Chicago Fox TV News - 'Immunizations - Are They Necessary'", CBC Newsworld Canada - "Are Mass Immunizations Necessary".

Since 1987, his weekly radio show "Family Health Forum", has aired in the Chicagoland area. In the live call-in format, all listener's comments, questions or medical experiences are welcome by Dr. Eisenstein.

Dr. Eisenstein's philosophy comes from his years in medicine, combined with his years as a husband, father, and grandfather (he has six children and six grandchildren).

Epilogue

In the months and the years to follow drug companies will come out with newer and better (sic) synthetic HRT drugs. Advertising that they are safer than the old ones. The market is huge, more than 20,000,000 women currently are taking synthetic HRT and the number of women becoming menopausal is growing at the rate of approximately 2,000,000 per year.

The newer SERMs (designer estrogens) and synthetic HRTs will promise you relief from multiple problems without any of the side effects of the previous estrogen drugs. Please view this in light of my favorite saying, drug companies do not let go of one drug until they find a more dangerous and profitable one to replace it.